Fallen Guardian Angels

Edward Ð Padilla

Acknowledgements

I extend my deepest gratitude to the following individuals who have helped contribute to "Fallen Guardian Angels"

Frank and Candy Padilla, Larry Chavez, Cheryl Pike-Vigil, Megan Pink, Theresa Roque-Dunaway, Robert Krzeksi, Ray Padilla, Cecilia Montero Marion Holeck, Claire Trautman, Rosendo Brown, James Baer Allen, David Yost, Sam Feuer, Charity Babcock-Jedeiken, Teddy Chen-Culver, Rosa Chavez, Jose Chavez, Elizabeth Taylor, Dr Thomas Church, Matt Chait, Tom Villard, Andrew Lauer, Lisa Rodriguez, Miss Dee, Patrick Buckham-Coleman, Ginger McCann, Alex Pink, Deven Ceriotti, Ani J. Darcey, Derek Alcaraz, Ryan Balint, Mayumi Koruda, Joel Castillo, EmLionel Marlon Bell, Jordan Bridges, Jacob Hollander, Timesha Congress, Lee Ludwig Meyers, Ace Charles Gilliam, Sean Patrick, David Ament, Beth Dandy, Abby Dandy, Marek Bute, Terry Skinner and Greg Nielson

ISBN: 978-0-615-50244-1

Sergius and Bacchus Publishing
New York, NY

10 9 8 7 6 5 4 3 2 1

Facebook.com/FallenGuardianAngelsLive - UnitedHopeProductions

Production inquiries: Edward_California@Yahoo.com

PRINTED IN THE UNITED STATES OF AMERICA

Cast of Characters:

STAGE MANAGER

AARON

HELEN

ROBERT

MARION

ROBIN

JARED

Setting: A theatre green room/dressing room.

Time: The time is May 1985

Fallen Guardian Angels

Fallen Guardian Angels

Act One

Setting: The dressing room/green room of a theatre. The set can be as minimal or elaborate as desired, as realistic or suggestive as needed, and as small or broad as effective. The essentials are six chairs, two small tables, a small tea cart with six wine glasses, one large martini glass, and a carafe of water, two lightweight trunks able to support the weight of two people sitting, six flameless candles, a phone, a small wastepaper basket, two wardrobe racks, a folded black sheet able to cover the two trunks when placed lengthwise to form a casket (the sheet also doubles as the "baby" in Aaron's scenes), and the colors: Red, Orange, Yellow, Green, Blue, and Purple. For effect, the set used in this script has a white cyclorama with color-changes to demonstrate the use of the colors. A small angel is 'hidden' in plain sight on the set.

At Rise: House lights at full, stage at half, and will remain this way until otherwise noted. The STAGE MANAGER, any sex, age, or race - enters. For simplicity, the Stage Manager will be referred to as "he". The Stage Manager places a vase of six roses, five red and one white, on one of the tables. He grabs his clipboard and places a few things for the characters (a serving tray near Jared's seat, etc.) He looks in one of the trunks and finds a flask. He pulls it out, takes a sip, and realizes the audience is watching him. He laughs nervously.

STAGE MANAGER

Caught me!

You know what? I believe in the illusion of theatre, but it's that fourth wall, I can't see you bullshit that bothers me. I see you! You! Hey! Youse on the phone. See you!

(He waits a moment)

As I said, kill the fourth wall. Okay, now, in 1981, maybe 1982, the first signs of the "gay cancer" hit our lives. How long ago was that? Right? Think about it, no one born after 1982 has ever lived in a world without this disease. Shit.

At the time, there was no cure. Hell, they didn't even know where it came from. Everyone knew that gay men got it, which really sucks, but the truth soon followed. Many people did not want to believe it, and many people still do not want to believe it, but it was not just a gay disease. Shortly, the C.D.C. announced two classifications: ARC, which stood for AIDS Related Complex, and AIDS. That's all we knew about it. Tada. ARC and AIDS. Oh, we knew that life expectancy was anywhere from three to six months, but that was it. Since then, breakthroughs in medicine help people live normal, long lives transforming AIDS from an automatic death sentence into a lifelong chronic disease.

Yeah. Yeah. This is a play. A piece of theatre. Like, "art". A docudramedy. I'm letting you know all this because "Fallen Guardian Angels" was written in May of 1985, three years into the epidemic. It was a time when we were still learning, still arguing, still wondering...still afraid.

STAGE MANAGER

(Continued)

These words have been heard around the world, helping people understand that, no matter how far we've come, we still have further to go. The playwright included information from over the years to add insight as to how things progressed...but, the story is still incomplete.

So, I take you back to the year "Fallen Guardian Angels" was first written.

(He waves his pen over audience)

Poof! I'm your fairy godmother. Member in good standing Mythical Creatures Union 748. Where the cyclops has his eye on you and the unicorns are always horny. Hoo-Rah!

> (Stage lights to full. House lights out. At this point, the performers are first seen. The characters are Aaron, male, mid-30s, Helen: female, early-50s, Robert: male, early-30s, Marion: female, mid-20s, Robin: female, late-20s, and Jared: male, late-30s. There are no ethnic requirements. There are various entrances that can be utilized: The actors can enter slowly from the back of the theatre and work their way up the aisle(s) toward the stage, or they can walk onto stage from the wings. If the performers are on stage, they should look downward and freeze into a position until noted. The actors are dressed in all black. Jared holds a small piece of paper.)

STAGE MANAGER

In 1985, there were no cell phones, so no one had to remind you to turn them off.

(He looks at the 'transgressor' from earlier)

The internet was just becoming the norm, and not many houses had computers.

Politically, Ronald Reagan sat in the White House, Soviet Leader Chernenko recently passed away, and Mikhail Gorbachev became their leader. Reagan and Gorbachev held a summit in November.

The San Francisco 49's won the SuperBowl against the Miami Dolphins. Bo Jackson won the Heisman Trophy. You know, if you're, like, into that sort of thing.

Feel like a night home? You could watch "The Golden Girls", "Family Ties" or "The Cosby Show." They came on once a week. You had to wait to see what would happen next.

At the movies, you could go see "Beverly Hills Cop" or "The Goonies" where a ticket cost you only three dollars. Yeah. That's right. Three dollars.

Now, the movie that interested me, in 1985, was "Back to the Future". Our Delorean just hit 88 miles per hour, so...welcome to our past.

> (The actors step out from behind the white curtains, or step onto the stage if entering from the theatre aisles. If they have been on stage, staring at the floor, they slowly look up and out over the audience)

STAGE MANAGER

Be thankful for the progress we've made to this point, but, in 1985, we had no idea what the future held.

!!!!!!

(The Stage Manager exits. The actors take the stage and begin preparing for their show. Please note each character's signature color: Aaron: red, Helen: Orange, Robert: Yellow, Marion: Green, Robin: Blue, Jared: Purple. The actors will NOT put on their signature color until their scene. Until then, they will remain in black. Jared will look at the paper in his hand. He crumples it and tosses it toward the wastepaper basket. He misses.)

AARON

Anyone have any extra eyeliner?

HELEN

(Hands some over)
Here you go, Aaron!

AARON

Thanks, Helen. I've been climbing the walls trying to find mine.

STAGE MANAGER (Off)

Five minutes! Five minutes to places.

ROBERT

Thank you, five!
(Searches)
Has anyone seen my hat for the second act?

HELEN
I thought it was under your table, sweetheart.

MARION
Or under Jared's.

ROBERT
Oh, sigh. That stud is straight.

ROBIN
Hallelujah! A straight man in theatre.

AARON
Two in this show.

JARED
Aaron? When you get a chance, we need to talk.

AARON
I'm free now.

JARED
After the show. I'm fighting butterflies right now.

HELEN
Opening night is so exciting.

ROBIN
Just pray your guardian angel doesn't fall.

MARION
What?

ROBIN

You get a guardian angel on the day you're born.

MARION

If you believe in that bullshit.

JARED

Some of us do.

ROBIN

Your guardian angel is there to protect you, keep you from harm. If your guardian angel fails, he falls. Please, God, let there be no fallen guardian angels tonight.

AARON

So everyone gets one of these guardian angels, even us Jews?

ROBIN

I believe so, yes.

AARON

Well, an angel is a terrible thing to waste.

HELEN

Be nice.

ROBERT

Jared? How did your doctor's appointment go today?

JARED

Doctor's appointment?

ROBERT
Remember? I saw you at...

JARED
Oh. Oh! No. I volunteer.

HELEN
Wonderful. Where?

JARED
Mercy Hospital.

ROBIN
Mercy?

HELEN
Ralph and Gary volunteer through a group there, too.

(A tense moment. Aaron stops, looking at Jared. Robin becomes uncomfortable. Helen crosses her arms, Robert's smile fades and Marion suddenly grabs her stomach)

MARION
Fuck a monkey. Why does my stomach hurt? I just had a good Mexican dinner.

JARED
There's some stomach stuff in the trunk, Marion.

MARION
Thanks, Jared.

ROBIN

Has anyone seen the crowd?

AARON

No, but I hope they laugh. I hate quiet crowds.
Happy, smiley people. Just laugh, dammit.

ROBERT

Sometimes, when they're quiet, I feel like the lights
are going to fall down on my head.

ROBIN

Drama queen.

JARED

Helen? Did Ralph show up?

HELEN

Second row.

STAGE MANAGER (off)

Two minutes! Two minutes!

AARON

Thank you, two!
          (Aaron will put on a red tie)

ROBERT

How's his boyfriend doing?

HELEN

Better. He hates being sick.

ROBERT

They're still together?

HELEN

Five years now.

JARED

Isn't that like the golden anniversary in gay years?

AARON

Gay dudes staying together that long. What a joke. They don't got no rights, no guarantees. One of them dies, the other loses everything.

HELEN

That's enough, Aaron. No arguing before we go on.

JARED

All we need is you and Robert going at it again.

ROBIN

Or him and Marion.

MARION

Hey! I haven't said crap about his closed-minded bullshit attitude.

AARON

I keep trying to tell you, Marion, lesbians are okay in my book. It's those faggots...

HELEN

Gays...

AARON

Gays that weird me out.

JARED

Weird you out?

AARON

Yeah. All they want is to have sex. No real commitment. Just sex.

HELEN

There are a lot of gay men who aren't just about the sex.

AARON

Not that many.

ROBERT

Like there aren't that many straight people who are about more than sex. Face it, Aaron, if there was a nice pair of titties in front of you...

AARON
(Interrupting)
Watch it, fag...gay. At least I know the difference between an entrance and an exit. Lesbians? Two entrances. Four with the out-doors. Six if they're willing.

MARION

Eat a dick, breeder.

AARON

Screw you, rug-muncher.

HELEN

Don't...please.

ROBERT

Fine! Fine! He's a breeder,
        (Points to Marion)
She's a lezbiatronic, and I'm a damn homo. Do we really have to go over this right now or can we just concentrate on doing a good show?

        (Aaron exits)

JARED

What is this fascination with some men and lesbians?

ROBIN

Jared, stop.

JARED

I always wondered about the fantasy.

HELEN

Jared!

JARED

Fine. Fine. Just trying to understand...

ROBIN
        (interrupting)
You should be trying to remember your lines.

JARED

I'll remember them.

STAGE MANAGER (off)

Places everyone! Places. Break a leg!

> (Aaron enters from side and stands center. All other performers are standing. These positions are essential for the end of act.)

AARON

My sister's sitting next to that damn homo...Homo's okay, right?   That homo that choreographed the fight scene.

ROBERT

You mean Brent?

AARON

Yeah, the fight guy. Always putting his arms around me.

ROBERT

He was trying to teach you how to pull a punch, sweetheart.

JARED

I feel sorry for him.

ROBIN

Sorry for him?

JARED

Yeah. He found out today he has AIDS.

ALL (Except Jared)

He has what?

(The actors, except AARON, will slowly sit in their chairs, and freeze into a 'signature pose'. They will remain in these poses unless otherwise directed. The less movement during the monologues, the better. The regular stage lighting will transition to Fantasy lighting as they sit. The light should focus on the forestage, where the monologues happen, and leave the non-speaking actors in dim-shadows. Each will say their line in a non-emotional manner:)

ROBERT

We would cruise the streets...

HELEN

When you hear a gay person is sick...

ROBIN

Why wasn't it me?

JARED

Nothing is forever.

MARION

Women don't get it.

(The actors are seated. We are now in Fantasy Lighting. Note: Unless "in scene", when actors speak during another actor's monologue, the 'interrupting' actor is to remain motionless and speak in a non-intrusive way. We are now in the minds of the actors. Everything is the form of a memory or dream.)

(Cyc to red: Cast in shadows)

AARON

You stood there, in a stark red dress against a red-brick wall. You wore a bright red hat. A big hat. Huge. You were decked out like you were going to church in Atlanta. You smiled at me with your big blue eyes piercing the walls around my heart, and I fell in love.

Was I supposed to know how it would end? Did you know the last time I would see you in that red dress would be the day they buried you? Did you mean to do this to me? Was I going to learn something?

How am I supposed to know what all this meant?

Answer me that. Before you came along, life was easy. Live life for the moment. I was young, selfish and insecure, but you changed that. Why did you change me?

I never asked *you* to change...but now I want...I want you to be like me. Alive. Alive and well. I want us to be together again so we can hold each other tightly after a great night making love. Watch the sun rise after a night of intense passion. Be there for each other as we conquer new goals.

Why did I ever care about you? What did you ever do for me?

You didn't come to my rescue when I needed you.

AARON

(Continued)

You were going to be a stronghold in my life. A life that needed your support. Where is it? Dammit!

You didn't give me the strength. You've given me nothing but despair. Not one ounce of hope is left in my heart...only despair.

Is that what it's supposed to be about? Is that what you meant by "love"?

Ha! Love.

I never loved anyone. I put up walls to keep me from that evil love. But you...you took the time to overcome my defenses and get to know the real me.

ROBIN

You are such a wonderful man. If only you could open up and talk to me. You have such strong walls.

AARON

If I let down my walls I'll be vulnerable.

ROBIN

We all take that chance, but sometimes it's worth it.

AARON

Will you share my walls?

ROBIN

Walls are meant to be torn down. Feelings are what we share.

AARON

I can't handle rejection.

ROBIN

I'm trying not to reject you. I really care.

AARON

I can't take that chance.

ROBIN

Let your defenses down...not me.

AARON

And you helped me tear them down. You made a home in my heart. You could do no wrong, even when you did wrong, you did no wrong. But you did lie to me.

You told me that bringing down my walls wouldn't hurt me. That people would get to know the real me and eventually love me. I didn't want to leave myself open like that. Open for people's judgments. Your judgment. But, because I love you, I left myself vulnerable.

You said no one would abandon me.

But you did..

What happened?

Why?

We lived together. Got married. Everything was so great...and, then...

But I kept fighting through. Went with you to counseling when we were dealt that bad hand. I did everything I could so I wouldn't lose you. I can't let you go. Don't you know I love you?

I was the luckiest man alive. Of all the people you could choose to wake up with; you chose me. How many others would give their right arm to be in my position? To see you

AARON

(Continued)

every day? To come home to you? To stand next to you as we washed dishes, watched television, sat on the lawn and had one of our backyard picnics?

I would never let you forget how much you mean to me. Never.

I bought you flowers. Roses that could never meet your beauty. Candy. Never to be as sweet as you.

ROBIN

Corny.

AARON

I know, but you always liked that lovey-dovey crap.

With all that, why is the only souvenir you kept of our life together a note? Not one flower pressed in a book. Not one piece of candy kept under your pillow...just a stupid note.

(Pulls 'note' out from pocket)

"Honey, you are the only reason for my life. I care about you and will miss you while you're away. If you feel any pain, call me. Day or night. I'm here for you. I love you. Aaron."

(puts note away)

I wrote that to you that day. The day you went to the hospital for what we thought was the last time. But you came home, better...and with a surprise. We were going to be a...

(Pause)

Pregnant?

ROBIN

Three months.

AARON

But what about...?

ROBIN

There's a less than eight percent chance I'll pass it on. He won't get it. He's too strong. He is our love.

AARON

A baby. I couldn't wait until we were a family. Nothing would ever separate us. Not one damn thing.

What happened?

After he was born...You were doing so well. Not once did I notice money missing from my wallet. Not once did I find a needle.

Why did you start using again?

(pause)

Did you remember to bleach your works?

Did you share a needle?

Then you got sick. Losing weight. Dehydrating.

But I was there. Me. Right there, by your side. You were in and out of the hospital so much, no one came to see you anymore. Yet, every day, where did you find me? Sitting in that god-awful brown plastic chair with the uneven chrome legs and cracked seat in the front that tore my jeans. Me. Right there, next to your hospital bed. I still don't understand why you didn't wait. You were my world. You promised me. You remember? I would not have to go through this alone...but now...

(Sound: Lullaby "All Through the Night" - soft and low. Helen and Robert stand and, mechanically, walk to the wardrobe, grab a surgical cap, mask, hospital gown and gloves and quickly dress Aaron in them. During this, Marion will grab the folded cloth and fashion it to look like a bundled baby. As soon as Aaron is dressed, Helen returns to her seat, Robert steps back, but does not sit. Marion hands the baby to Aaron before returning to her seat. Sound: Lullaby ENDS)

AARON

Honey, our baby...little Shawn...turns three next month...If he makes it. They have him on so many machines at Mercy Hospital that I can't look at him sometimes. He looks like he's in so much pain.

(Pulls down surgical mask)

Do I really need all this crap?

ROBERT

We must take necessary precautions to keep others from getting sick.

AARON

But he's just a baby.

(Robert pulls out a vial of pills from pocket. He hands them to Aaron. He pulls Aaron's surgical mask over Aaron's mouth.)

ROBERT

Remember to crush two of these pills into his applesauce in the morning. One of the yellow pills dissolved into his formula twice a day. Two drops of the brown liquid every night one half hour before he goes to sleep.

(returns and sits)

AARON

(Pulls surgical mask down. To audience.)

How in the hell am I supposed to know when he's going to sleep? I don't even know when I'm going to sleep until I find myself...well...asleep.

It's a lot to remember, just like you reminded me...Yes...I know...I've been baptized plenty of times in the name of father-son urine, but I don't mind.

Holding him is holding you, and I would give anything to hold you again. To come home to your bright, blue-eyed smile.

Now I come home and stand in an empty nursery looking at a lonely crib with those soft sheets and that thirty-inch thick comforter...God, you agonized for weeks over buying that damn thing. All those months looking through books and catalogues.

We were going to be Norman Rockwell dipped in a hazy buzz.

I can still smell your perfume mixing with the baby powder.

All that planning, and our baby...our little Shawn...he'll never see it. He'll never rest his head on your grandmother's handmade needlepoint pillow. He'll never bundle in that comforter.

AARON

(Continued)

What a fucking waste.

> (He unfurls the blanket...clutching one corner in his hand.)

I used to think AIDS was just a gay disease, not for straight people like you and me. Shawn's only three. He never had a chance to determine his lifestyle. Where's the truth now? Where can justice be found by a three-year-old baby? He is the only living memory I have of you, and he's leaving me.

I can't go on. He is us, and our love is dying.

> (Tosses blanket to the ground.)

But when I look into his eyes, I see your hope. Your determination. He is the only person I've ever known who loves without boundaries. He doesn't have to break through my walls...I never put any up for him.

> (Pulls off surgical 'gear' and throws it under the wardrobe rack.)

He doesn't deserve this. He deserves to be held. He deserves to feel his father's hands, his father's arms, his father's breath.

He doesn't deserve anything but love.

> (Lovingly gathers up blanket from the ground.)

You are flesh of my flesh, and love of my love. I will hold you. I promise I will touch you. I promise you will not know a day without feeling my arms around you. I promise you because I am determined that your short time on this earth will be filled with love, not isolation.

AARON

(Continued)

And maybe...just maybe...Shawn will see my struggle. Maybe Shawn will see my determination, and he'll try harder.

He's a natural-born fighter.

And he'll fight.

Fight?

He's only three, dammit. Only three. He shouldn't have to fight.

Take me. Leave the children alone. They didn't hurt anyone.

They are our future.

And our future is dying.

(Aaron will put the cover back where it was originally found. During the next few lines, before they are completed, he will hang up the hospital gown and other paraphernalia, but leave on his red tie. He will sit in his chair and assume his signature pose.)

(Cyc to white. Cast in half light.)

ROBIN

How did this whole thing start?

MARION

On June fifth, 1981, the Center for Disease Control, the C.D.C., reports that in the period from October 1980 through May of 1981, five young men, all active homosexuals, were treated for biopsy-confirmed Pneumocystis Carinii Pneumonia at three different

MARION

(Continued)

hospitals in Los Angeles, California. Two of the patients died.

ROBERT

On July fourth, 1981, the C.D.C. reports that during the past thirty months there were twenty-six diagnosed cases of Kaposi Sarcoma among gay males, and that eight have died, all within two years of diagnosis.

ROBIN

Kaposi Sarcoma? That's a disease found only in cats. It's a cluster of Bartonella bacteria, the same organisms that causes Cat Scratch disease.

ROBERT

It's most outward sign is dark lesions...splotches...on the skin.

(Helen will put on an article of orange.)

JARED

With all the buzz spreading about this new disease, President Ronald Reagan does not use the word AIDS.

ROBERT

Trying to remove the "gay-only" misinformation about the disease, in 1982, the C.D.C. changes the name of this new disease from GRIDS...The "G" standing for 'gay'...to AIDS.

ROBIN

But where did AIDS come from?

JARED

Biological Warfare.

MARION

Someone fucked a monkey.

AARON

It's a punishment from God!

ROBIN

Dammit all to hell. People, where did it start?

ROBERT

No one knows.

ROBIN

If no one knows how it started, then where do we go
from here?

(Cyc to Orange: Cast in shadows)

HELEN

My son Ralph is my pride and joy, the love of my
life, the reason for my existence, and he's gay.

That's right. Gay.

He's a homo.

Got a problem with that? I didn't think so.

He lives with his lover, Gary, in a two-bedroom
condo that they bought. Bought. Well, of course,
everyone knows that homosexuals make great gobs

HELEN

(Continued)

of money, they have money falling out of their...let's just say wallets, okay? If the bulge in the back doesn't match the bulge in the front. Well, if women worried as much about a man's size as gays do, none of us would have ever been born. What is it that Ralph said? Oh! More than a mouthful is a waste. Less than a mouthful? Not even a taste.

You know, back in my day, we didn't talk this openly about sex. It was taboo. Something you did behind closed doors. Even television programs had married couples sleeping in separate beds. I'm surprised they were in the same room.

Nowadays, well...I saw this show on television, network of all things, and this young man's rear end was right there for everyone to see. I couldn't believe it. I was glad I recorded it so I could make sure I saw exactly what I thought I saw, and I did. I was so upset that I called my friend, Clarice, and she came over to watch, and even she didn't believe it. Now she comes over every Wednesday, and we haven't missed an episode since.

But it shows you how much things have changed. At one time, you couldn't even think about saying "damn" on stage. You could drink tap water. You didn't have to wear seatbelts. Now...Ralph and Gary told me they just bought a new car. Zero to sixty in six seconds. Lordy! Back in my day, cars only reached sixty on a good decline.

And shame on you if you believe that. I'm not that old, dammit.

HELEN

(Continued)

People. People love to go fast. Ralph and Gary? Not that fast. Took it nice and slow, and now they have one beautiful relationship.

They love each other. They communicate. That's what today's relationships need: Communication. That's why Ralph knew it was okay to tell me he's gay. Communication. We left those lines open to each other's hearts. He could tell me anything. And I told him to remember the rules of love. No matter who you love; first you meet, do some courting, get married, and then you have a baby.

The day my water broke...

(The Cast collectively drops their heads - They've heard this before)

I went into the delivery room and they put my feet up in the stirrups and told me Ralph was on his way. That was the most exciting day of my life. Through the pain...I struggled. I pushed. I breathed. My husband relaxed in the waiting room and smoked a pack of Lucky Strikes.. Finally, Ralph's little head...

(coughs)

...appeared, shoulders, and then Ralph came into this world. I saw the most perfect little boy, covered in blood and slimy crap and crying like the dickens...but all I could say was, "I love you."

(Cast back to signature poses)

I loved him every day since, and my love only grows stronger.

And you mamas out there? And you daddies, too. If your child comes to you and tells you they're gay, remember the day you held your child in your arms for the first time...You loved your child then,

HELEN

(Continued)

and probably promised nothing bad would ever happen to them. Keep your promise. The world can be a hateful place, and they'll learn that eventually. Don't let them learn hate from you. No matter what. Let them know love, and remind them for every one person that hates you, there are one hundred people that love you. It's true even for you. Right now, as you're sitting here, someone out there...someone you don't even know...loves you. Make sure you know that, and make sure your children know it, too. Don't be their first bad memory.

And love is so wondrous and beautiful. Those first moments...those last moments...When Ralph met Gary, he first courted him. They committed to each other a few months later, and then they moved in together a year after that. Then they bought a puppy.

(Resigned.)

That's *my* grand-baby. They call him Poppers. Little Poppers.

Oh, I'm not that dumb. I know that poppers are an Amyl-Nitrate base inhalant for temporary highs, but that mutt isn't much of a danger. He can give you a headache like those poppers can.

What? You don't think I'm an educated woman? When this crap started about AIDS, and people screamed that poppers spread this disease, well, I didn't believe it. I decided to find out for myself. What was in that magical little brown bottle that caused AIDS?

Well, I walked right into that adult bookstore three blocks from Ralph and Gary's condo...What is the

HELEN

(Continued)

name of it? Oh, I can't remember. It's right on the tip of my tongue. It's either Pussycat or Kitty-Titties. Something like that. I saw they had them poppers, so I put my money on the counter and bought some.

When I took it home...I inhaled.

Wooh! The head rush! And the feeling. It wasn't anything like having a good size joint to yourself, and it didn't last that long.

(The rest of the cast slowly look toward her) Sort of like getting some skunk when you think you're getting the primo shit...

I mean...Hell, if you want to get a little quicky rush, those poppers will do.

(All back to original positions)

I still have not caught the AIDS. Unless it's hiding in the liquid, you cannot catch it from there, and, even then, you'd have to get it into your blood. I'll admit it makes you a little horny and ready to jump on anything and ride it like Mariah, but...we can be responsible adults, right?

Look at you all staring at me like I'm crazy. So what if I experiment? So what if I want to dress up like Wonder Woman and tie my husband in my golden lasso and torture him until he talks? I want to live this life to the fullest and have no regrets. If I'm considered crazy for getting my nipples pierced last Thursday, then so be it. I couldn't wear a bra for three days, but I feel alive.

Call me the bad girl if you want. The rest of my family is what you would consider normal. Good. Me? It's hard to believe Ralph is as calm as he is.

HELEN

(Continued)

Takes after his father. And Ralph and Gary are good boys. They really are. I haven't seen a relationship as strong as theirs.

Oh, don't get me wrong. They fight. Lordy, some of the fights they have. When Ralph had to miss Gary's college graduation...oh, my word...The fight lasted for days. Ralph's job required him to go out of town that week. Well, graduation is important. They said things to each other that made the puppy cringe. Oh, yeah, they should have broken up, but they didn't because those lines of communication were open. They learned to talk it out after the yelling. They learned it wasn't indignant to say I'm sorry. To forgive. To move forward. I guess more people need to learn that. More than that, people need to grow a sense of humor. If my husband and I weren't able to laugh, I'd have belted him in the mouth more than once.

(Loud sneeze)

Excuse me.

I think I'm catching a cold. God, I hate being sick.

Ralph came to me today and told me that Gary was sick.

ROBERT

I'll be there tonight, mom, but Gary's going to miss it. He has a fever.

HELEN

Are you okay?

ROBERT
I think so. I'm not showing any symptoms.

HELEN
Make sure you wear a condom, and use lots and lots of lube. The AIDS virus is known to pass through semen because of rips in the colon. You have to be careful, baby. I don't want you to die.

ROBERT
Mom! Seriously? He has the flu. You hear a gay man is sick and you immediately think AIDS?

HELEN
       (To audience)
We all do. Don't deny it. We hear a gay man is sick and we think AIDS. It's got to be AIDS.

   Don't lie to yourself. Probably comes from our deep fear of homosexuality. And those news reporters telling us every night that AIDS is found only in the gay community.

   We make gays the scapegoats. We are afraid of them, so it's alright to say they're the only people who get this AIDS thing. God forbid you see two men touching. Holy shit-on-a-shingle, that's just not done.

   In today's society, it is unseen for two men to hug, kiss, feel. They are too masculine for that sort of thing. Why? It isn't degrading to love someone. That's the highest compliment you can give a

HELEN
(Continued)

person. Whether they're of the same sex or not, that's not the point.

Everyone's afraid to touch each other. Oh, sure, it's easier to touch yourself...not like that...okay, maybe like that. It is safer than just jumping into bed with someone. But we need to learn how to touch with a feeling of adequacy, not inadequacy. If you're strong enough to take a person to bed, be strong enough to let that person see you for who you really are. Don't just have sex. With all those diseases out there, if you need to just have sex, then...Yes! Learn a form of self-service. It's safe and easy...unless your batteries die. But women can make allowances...You think God shaped a banana that way on accident?

If you really need someone else, then show who you really are. Take care...use precautions.

Whoops! Where's my soapbox? I didn't come here for that.

Did I tell you about my husband, John? He died a little over a year ago.

I'm going to tell you this: Be proud of who you love. Tell who you want. But...never...never ever never...tell your father you're gay while he's trying to maneuver a tricky turn on the highway at sixty-five miles an hour. We're not sure if he had a heart attack or...point is...choose the right spot and the right time.

God, I miss him.

We had some wonderful years together. That's the truth. When I heard he died, I grieved. It was part of my acceptance. I took those five steps to allowing myself to say John is dead. But I think we need a new

HELEN

(Continued)

step in that process. Death. Grieving. First you're in denial. This is not true. It cannot be true. Then there's anger. Rage. How can this be happening? Bargaining. If I do this, then this will happen. Then there's depression...sadness...and we finally come to acceptance. Five stages. Boom! We're supposed to be back to...ahem...normal. But I ask you, shouldn't we add forgiveness to the pot? Before we accept the end, shouldn't we forgive? Say I'm sorry? Or, at least, say it's not your fault? It's not my fault?

Forgiveness. Food for thought.

John was always afraid of the dark, so Ralph and I agreed on cremation. Why stick the love of my life in some dark hole underground?

Me? I'm not afraid of nothing. Not the dark, not tight spaces, and definitely not what other people think of me. It's my life, and, when it's over, I want to know I lived for me. And when I die, I want to be cremated and have my ashes placed in an urn and put on Ralph and Gary's mantel. They always bring me joy when they're around. They remind me so much of John and myself.

They'll last. They've learned.

And I just love it when Gary snaps his fingers and calls me "Girlfriend!"

(Helen sits, leaving on her orange.)

(Cyc to white. Cast in half light.)

ROBIN

The number of known AIDS related deaths in the U.S.A. in 1982 is 853. In 1983 it's 2304. In 1984 it's 4251. Gaetan Dugas, listed as "Patient Zero" in *And The Band Played On,* was one of the people who died in 1984.

ROBERT

Gaetan Dugas had that notorious title removed from him in 1995, when it was discovered he was used only as a fictional plot-point. Scientists begin learning the nexus of AIDS started long before we heard about it.

JARED

Ronald Reagan still refuses to use the word AIDS. He doesn't acknowledge it. If the president ignores this, people will ignore it, too.

AARON

The highest percentage of AIDS related deaths is gay people. Straights feel they have nothing to worry about. For all they know, it won't affect them.

JARED

Really?

AARON

According to the C.D.C., sixty percent, that's two out of every three, of all AIDS cases went unreported between 1981 and 1990. Many of them were heterosexuals because they were afraid people would think they're gay.

(Robert puts on an article of yellow clothing)

JARED
It's time for people to learn, but I don't know how to start. Where do we go from here?

(Cyc to yellow. Cast in shadows.)

ROBERT
(Directed to audience)
But how is he?

ROBIN
I cannot disclose that information.

ROBERT
Last time I spoke to him, he had a viral load of 750,000 and a T-Cell count of forty-two.

ROBIN
I cannot deny or confirm this. You're not his real family.

ROBERT
Look, you arrogant shit-for-brains, he's my baby brother.
  You know him as Patient Z-2-1-6-2-0-6-1-1.
  His name is Vince.
  I call him "Bitch". He is a vivacious, caring and outgoing person. When we met, AIDS was a tiny word that didn't scare anyone. We saw nothing wrong with hopping from cruise bar to porn shop to bath house.

ROBERT

(Continued)

And we had sex. Lots of it. Few tricks had names. Hell, some didn't even have faces. We saw love as a joke. Sex? A bet. "I can get more dick than you can" was *the* catchphrase of the day.

You didn't talk about condoms. Those were for sissies. If you didn't have the clap...gonorrhea...it was "hold his legs in the air, because I'm halfway there."

(Softer)

I am standing in front of you with mixed emotions...Why? Because someone I know, someone every dear to me, asked me to talk to you. He wanted me to tell you how he's changed since he's caught AIDS.

That is impossible to do without telling you what he was like before he caught the disease.

Vince and I met years ago. We remain friends to this day.

We had the same insatiable need for sex. And we would find a guy, and...well....Let's just say that the game, "Tag", took on a new meaning.

I remember those times dearly. Vince and I would cruise the streets at night, looking for studs lurking in the yellow glow of the streetlamps.

JARED

There's one.

ROBERT

Too young.

JARED

As if.

ROBERT

Slap a boutonniere on the bitch and take him to prom.

JARED

Him!

ROBERT

Braces.

(Robert puts his hands over his crotch as...)

JARED and ROBERT

Ewww...

JARED

Over there.

ROBERT

Now you're talking.

And like wolves stalking a helpless buck, we'd pounce on him in a frenzy of unmitigated lust.

Damn it was fun. Real fun. And Vince and I shared those times. He helped me accept me...helped me be me. I guess I never thanked him for that.

Then there was a two year absence from each other. A lot can happen in two years, and it did.

For one, I went back in the closet. This AIDS thing was hitting the gay community, and hitting it hard, And, as a gay man, I was part of that community. I didn't see friends anymore, and when I snuck out to

ROBERT
(Continued)
the bar...I found out I wouldn't see some friends ever again.

I stopped having sex. Blasphemy! But I did.

And, then, one night, he walked back into my life.

When I first saw Vince, he was trying to be the same person he used to be. Cracking jokes, doing dish and swish...flaming.

But there was something different to him. Falseness. A cover. His smiled seemed forced. He was searching for something, maybe trying to find his lost youth.

I was so excited to see him. I ran up, arms spread, big smile, and...You know what Bitch's first words were to me? "Nice to see you." To hell with that. "Nice to see you?" Yeah..."Nice to see you." You say that to a politician. You say that to a great aunt you want to make sure keeps you in the will. You do not say "nice to see you" to a guy you've helped slide down on a nine inch... (cock).

JARED
(interrupting)
Let's not talk about it, okay?

ROBERT
Not talk about it?

JARED
It's who I was, not who I am.

ROBERT
And who are you now?

JARED

Different. Same person, just...I've changed.

ROBERT

What's wrong?

JARED

Nothing. Missed you.

ROBERT

You're about as choked up about missing me as you'd be about missing freaking "Murder She Wrote". Tell me the truth. What's wrong?

JARED

I have it.

ROBERT

It?

JARED

It.

ROBERT

The disease. You know the one. That disease they whisper about in the back room of the bar.

How? Why?

Vince had changed. He wasn't "happy-come-fuck-me" anymore. He became very emotional, and apt to mood swings.

Severe mood swings.

He had changed all right, and not for the better. What could possibly make a person change that

ROBERT
(Continued)

much? Death? Helplessness? What? Everything that Vince could be feeling came swimming into my head.

MARION

Don't touch me!

AARON

We need separate water fountains and bathrooms.

HELEN

Know the wrath of God punishing you for your sins.

ROBERT

Man, the crap he must be going through. Not some of it, but all of it.

I had to wonder how I would handle it. You know what? Not half as good as him.

I had to admire his courage. He laughed it off. He did his best to make us unaware of his...um...his word, not mine...misfortune.

You just *know* we had to relive our tradition by banging a twinkie. A twinkie. You know what I mean: Fresh, young, creams when you squeeze him.

As we methodically seduced our young stud into a need for sex matched only by his need for air; Vince slowly encased his erect member in a condom lubricated with spermicide.

Okay. Honestly? The first time I tasted that latex sheath...I gagged, and not in the good way. I didn't feel like I was doing a human. It was like sucking on a pacifier. Rubber. No one could enjoy this. But

ROBERT

(Continued)

Vince leaned my head up from our prey's hot instrument, and I watched as my mouth drove my idol to a burst of passion. I never knew an orgasm could be so fantastic for both parties.

And the best part?

No cock breath!

Vince taught me a lot that night. He taught me a lot about myself, too. Sure, I had grown up, but I never took life for what it was.

Life is a precious gift. A gift I take for granted every day.

Vince makes every day count. He doesn't have much time left. Very little time. We all think we have this long, long life ahead of us...we'll get to it later...but Vince? He's all out of "later".

Oh, sure. I know we all have the chance of getting hit by the obligatory bus while crossing cliché street, but no one ever thinks about that. But waking up every day facing your own death? Well, that day becomes very special.

Someone holding your hand becomes special.

Yes, Vince can be very forgetful at times, and he can get on your nerves because you never know what mood he'll be in, but he's become insightful. Watching him, I learned condoms can be used in erotic ways. Sex doesn't have to kill you. It can be fun again.

And love? Just because I treated love like a joke...it didn't mean I didn't want it.

I love Vince, but we're tried and true...brothers above others.

ROBERT

(Continued)

He's given up on love...But he hasn't given up on him...

When I first met Vince, he was strong. Now he's stronger in a *positive* way. He's become a fighter. He stands up for himself. He will not let this stupid disease get the best of him. He's become the type of person I would love to be.

She's butch.

(Snaps fingers)

Truth is...he's become a true-true friend.

And friends are there for each other, good times and bad. You care for each other. You support each other. You help each other get laid.

And, despite all the changes he's gone through...we've gone through...there's one thing that hasn't changed.

He's my friend.

My little brother.

I'll miss him when he's gone, but I thank God for him while he's still here.

(Robert crosses to his seat leaving on his yellow)

(Cyc to white. Cast in half light.)

ROBIN

I heard the biggest news of 1985 was the F.D.A. finally approved the first AIDS antibody test for blood. The U.S.A. and Japan begin testing their blood products.

JARED

In 1985, our 'fearless' commander in chief, Ronald Reagan finally did use the word "AIDS" in an off-handed remark when responding to reporters' questions.

AARON

1985 was a big year in numbers. The number of AIDS related deaths in the U.S.A. that year was 5636.

(Marion puts on a green article of clothing)

HELEN

On October second, 1985, Rock Hudson died from AIDS. This was the start of the "maybe straights can get it" mentality because many people...many, many people, believed Rock Hudson was straight. I didn't care. Straight or gay, in my fantasies; he did things to me that...well, I loved him in "Giant" with James Dean...But if he were alive today...I know what we'd be doing right now.
        (Fans herself)
Is it hot in here?
        (Fans her crotch)
I know it's humid. Oh, Rock, come to me!

AARON

And she's off...
        (guiding Helen back to her seat)
It's too bad he's dead, right?

(Cyc to Green. Cast in shadow)

ROBIN

Denial.

MARION

It's just cancer.

It is the duty of everything in nature to survive. Survival of the fittest and all that. You taught me that. You'll beat it. It's not even malignant. You're stronger than cancer. You are my heart. You are the strong one.

ROBIN

I have complications from AIDS.

MARION

Stop lying to me. Just stop.

Survival of the fittest is the key to the cycle of nature. When something dies, nature uses it, recycles it, and keeps the circle going.

A field mouse, after dying, feeds thousands of maggots. These maggots metamorphasize... Metamorphicate...

(Frustrated)

Change into flying insects and pollinate plants. Plants provide oxygen for animals and food for the field mouse. It's a never-ending circle in the survival of nature. Everything works together.

Everything except for man, that is.

Man is a parasite. Digging, using, abusing and taking. You know what happens when all you do is take and never give anything back? It all dries up. There isn't anything left.

Man rapes the forest, kills the trees, and then uses those oxygen-creating goddesses to create paper on

MARION

(Continued)

which they print pictures and numbers and give it value. Money.

But we don't value the trees.

When did man become irresponsible in the eyes of the animals? When did man become the parasites? Why are they a virus on this planet when we could be a cure?

We should apologize to our Mother Earth, and earn her respect back. That's what my love, my heart, Nicole, always tells me. She takes Botany down at the university. She was *in* to nature. She wanted to live in a cave, commune with the environment. Eat oat bran. You know, I don't think she was irregular once in her life.

Oh, don't get me wrong. She is still alive, but she needs help. She's dying of cancer.

ROBIN

And I have complications from AIDS.

MARION

Stop.

Nicole and I met three years ago, and we have what you'd call an open relationship because she is bi. That ugly third leg turned her on. One time, she had me strap on this...

Never mind. Not important.

But she liked men. I asked her if she was careful, and she told me that she always wore her I.U.D. and she only sleeps with straight men. Then how can she get this disease? It's a fag disease. No one gets it but homos and Haitians.

MARION

(Continued)

That's how I know she's lying. Cancer will do that to a person, know what I mean? People find out they're sick so they add more diseases to themselves for attention and pity. I won't pity you.

Lesbians do not get AIDS.

HELEN

Denial.

MARION

How can anyone believe she has it? Are they that dumb? Women aren't carriers. Women do not have sperm.

I heard you can catch AIDS from fucking a monkey, and, well, Nicole would just not *do* that.

Then how?

Psychosomatic.

JARED

Denial.

MARION

All in the brain. She even has the doctors convinced. They took her blood and they found AIDS. It has to be a false positive. You can have those, you know. Or maybe...maybe they mixed her blood up with someone else's. Mistakes happen, and Nicole always told me that a human's first mistake is that they're human. It's totally downhill after that.

Nicole wanted another test. That was her first mistake.

MARION

(Continued)

ELISA. The Enzyme-Linked Immuno Sorbent Assay test. ELISA looks specifically for the AIDS antibodies and is eighty-six to ninety percent accurate, but there's still a chance for error.

AARON

Denial.

MARION

That's why she wants another freaking test. This one is called "The Western Blot." It's a test that will specifically search for the AIDS virus.

She cannot have it, and she's spending all this money trying to prove she does. How dare her!

Another test? Babe, my heart, these tests aren't cheap.

ROBIN

I need to know. Don't you want to know?

MARION

But...you're a woman...My heart, my love...Women don't get this.

ROBIN

I love you. If you love me, then please...

MARION

For you, then, anything. But you'll see…

AARON

Unified Insurance does not cover AIDS-related
treatment.

MARION

It's only cancer.

ROBIN

Denial.

MARION

You know what's the truth? These treatments and
tests aren't cheap.

I saved up some money and had the doctors test
me for AIDS. You know what they found? Nothing!
Do you hear me? Negative. I'm a woman, and
women don't get AIDS.

JARED

Denial.

MARION

Cancer. That's all she has. Nicole is making it
worse by pretending to have AIDS. Her world of
make believe is going to end. It has to. Face the truth.
I've always told her that. Face the truth.

Why are you trying to make me believe her lies?
She has a cage around her that is stopping her from
more glorious things.

(The following must be staccato and fast)

HELEN

Face the truth.

MARION

Nicole can't have AIDS. She's a woman.

JARED

See the truth.

MARION

Only homosexuals get AIDS.

AARON

You can't lie to yourself.

MARION

I don't have it. How can she?

ROBERT

Tell yourself the truth because it isn't survival to lie to your soul.

MARION

There's no way in hell she can have it. Not my Nicole.

Nicole would not sleep with anyone but a straight man or me. No one would lie to her about having AIDS. Maybe there was a straight man out there that used a dirty needle.

No. That wouldn't happen.

But, if he did, he could lie. Maybe he was infected, and he gave it to Nicole.

There's no way. She wouldn't allow that. She was careful. Really careful. She would not let herself sleep with a man that has AIDS. She'd never do that.

Nature. Survival of the fittest.

MARION

(Continued)
Nicole's fit.
    She'll never die.

(Sits, leaving on her green.)

(Cyc to white. Cast in half-light)

HELEN

The term ARC, three little letters, is changed by the
Center for Disease Control to HIV in 1987, and
finally consider people with HIV part of the AIDS
statistic.

JARED

On April second, 1987, with virtually no mention at
all, President Reagan appears before the College of
Physicians in Philadelphia to give his first 'major
speech' on AIDS, calling it "Public Enemy Number
One".

AARON

And his vice president, George Bush, gets heckled
when he cries for mandatory HIV testing.

JARED

Three years later, 1990, Ronald Reagan apologizes
for his neglect of the epidemic while he was
president.

ROBERT

Okay, enough Reagan bashing. Remember, federal
anti-AIDS spending grew dramatically throughout

ROBERT

(Continued)

Reagan's term. The eight million dollars that Reagan approved in 1982 rocketed to two-point-three billion dollars in 1989. The average annual increase in federal funding for AIDS research under Reagan was basically 129 percent per year. Yes, he ignored saying anything about AIDS, but he didn't ignore needed funding. Can't you say anything positive about AIDS history?

JARED

Thomas Netter and James W. Bunn of the World Health Organization come up with the idea of World AIDS Day in 1987. In 1988, an election year...

(Robert clears throat)

The first World AIDS Day is celebrated on December first in 1988...

(Quick aside)

...an election year...

World AIDS Day events begin to grow every year after that. December becomes AIDS Awareness month in 1990.

ROBERT

The number of known AIDS related deaths in the U.S. in 1990 is 18,477, including Ryan White, born December 6, 1971. He was a teenager and AIDS activist who went to heaven on April eighth. Terrible how so many great people are just a statistic now.

AARON

And he was straight.

MARION

Straight men don't get it.

JARED

Everyone can get it.

MARION

Everyone?

JARED

Everyone.

MARION

But...

(Robin puts on a blue preacher's stole)

HELEN

You know, the first step toward a new future is always found at a choice. Either decision will lead to a different outcome. Which direction do we go? We stand on the base of a mountain and can only wonder, where do we go from here?

(Lights on main area)

(Cyc to Blue. Cast in shadows.)

ROBIN

We go to God. We trust in God. Praise the lord, for He has given us many glorious things! Pray with me.

ROBIN
(Continued: The rest bow their heads)
Dear Lord, let my words comfort as well as educate
this congregation. Amen.

ALL
Amen.

ROBIN
Hallelujah! I was raised a good girl. Never wore my
skirts too high or my shoes too shiny. I prayed every
morning...every evening. I especially prayed before
going to bed...why? Because the bible says that
death is a thief in the night, and I wanted to be ready.

Lord! Take me from this humble existence. I am
tired of it.

But I wasn't bad enough. So, I let my free will take
over. I turned to alcohol! Lucifer's liquid! Started
doing drugs! No, not the needly kind, just the devil's
weed! Pot and pills and drinks without spills. I
became sexually active. Slept with whoever I
wanted to. Male.
(Cups side of mouth: Secret)
Female.
(Normal)
Let's face it. I was easy. Living for the lord in
unrighteous accord.

There wasn't a lotion or position I didn't try.

I could eat a foot-long hot dog without leaving a
bite mark.

Got your attention...

ROBIN

(Continued)

My nickname in high school was Winnie Bago, because I could easily sleep twelve.

So, let me ask you something. Why didn't I get sick? Why didn't I get AIDS? I heard it was a punishment from God for living a sinful life.

I'm still well.

Where's my punishment?

I should be lying in a bed, tubes running out every God-made and man-made hole in my body, and getting those 'down-your-nose' uppity-bitch looks from everyone.

You know who gets them looks?

My brother.

Brian.

Let me tell you, he never did nothing wrong. He stayed away from drugs...He cut the grass, he didn't smoke it. Stayed away from alcohol...He even stayed away from sex...He was waiting until he got married to have sex. Can you believe it? A twenty year old virgin. Seriously. Twenty years old and never had sex..

Oh, and he prayed. Hell, he prayed more than me. He is good. Purely good.

How, then, could he get a disease that's for the ungodly people of the world?

That's what everyone says, right? AIDS is a punishment from God for living a sinful life. It fits his M.O., you know? I mean, God destroyed Sodom and Gomorrah for screwing around. God even had the nerve to toss Adam and Even out of Paradise just for eating some stupid apple.

ROBIN

(Continued)

One thing for sure, God knows how to punish people.

But...wait...Famed preachers of the world, National T.V. evangelists are sleeping around, and they're not sick. God makes me angry with His inconsistencies. Why God be loving on those greedy bastards but hating on my brother?

Where is the justification? Where is the righteousness?

Maybe we need to stop believing that God punishes the unjust.

No. No. No. No. Hell, no.

People always need to believe in an artfully vengeful God. That way they can be spreading their hate in the name of the Lord. Then, on Sunday, they tell themselves that God loves them and no one else. You know what? It's peoples' inconsistencies pissing me off.

If God hates us, He hates all of us. If God loves us, He loves all of us.

Let's go with the love. You know why? Because God so loved the world that He gave us his only Son to die for the sinners. Why would God send Jesus to die for the perfect ones? I didn't read in no bible how Jesus said, "Okay, check it out. I'm dying for the forgiveness of sins, but not of the sins of these people, or those people, or especially not those people." Jesus said he was dying for all of us...saints and sinners alike. Now, that's some loving right there.

ROBIN

(Continued)

Why, then, are people saying that God is punishing us with this disease? Something inherently good would be continually good.

I guess people don't believe in their God anymore. Why not?

They sure believe in Him when they need him. Please, God, don't let me wreck in this rain. Please, God, let me find a job. Please, God, let this be the winning lottery ticket. But, damn sure if they don't forget Him the minute their hate wants to take control. God hates fags, that's why he gave them AIDS.

Let me ask you something. I've been upfront with you. My brother, Brian? He doesn't do drugs. Brian doesn't have sex. Brian doesn't do anything risky...no big boners up the bung or sticking the skin. He lives a completely...how do I put this? He lives..."good".

So, answer me this: Why does my brother have AIDS?

(Pause: Cast looks at Robin - Give this a ten count)

Brian was in a car accident.

(Cast back to signature poses)

Brian was hurt. Badly hurt. He needed surgery. During surgery, he needed blood. A transfusion. Now, according to the hospital, the blood was properly processed and did not carry the AIDS virus. It must have made it through a window.

Do you know what 'properly processed' means? It means that for every 1000 pints of blood they get, the place that takes the blood only has to test ten.

ROBIN

(Continued)

Ten. Basically one out of every hundred bags of blood is tested for the AIDS virus.

If one bag in one hundred is good, they are all considered good.

That's one hell of a big window.

But now you know. My brother, the saint that he is, got the sinner's disease because someone else was trying to save money.

Sort of screws with the whole "God is punishing us" mentality.

I'll tell you this much, God ain't punishing Brian, but those people at the hospital treat him like he's a criminal.

When I go to see him, I hear them call him Three-Forty-One-Two. Room 341...that's Brian's room...and he's in bed two. They call him everything but "Brian". He's just a number, a statistic, a paycheck. They treat him like crap.

Me? Oh, they treat me like gold. I'm not a sinner...I don't got AIDS, you see.

Why, hello...How'm I doing? Well, I was sucking your husband's dick five minutes before I came in here, Nurse Sunshine...but I'm fine.

HELEN

Ahem.

ROBIN

To them, Brian's the sinner, because of someone else's mistake.

Talk about compassion.

ROBIN

(Continued)

How can anyone, anyone at all, believe this is a punishment from love? It can't be. Logically. Think about it. If you loved someone, would you want to see that person in pain? Would you, if you loved someone, want to give them something that would kill them?

If you would, then you don't love that person...Do you?

You know who wants to inflict pain?

People with hate in their heart. Dark souls. They're the ones who want to destroy other people. They are so sorry-ass fed up with their own pathetic lives, that they cause confusion and chaos. They do everything they can to destroy the other person.

And if God is the purest example of love; then Satan, or the devil, would be the purest example of hate, and hate wants to cause destruction.

Destruction isn't just destroying lives, but destroying character, destroying compassion.

So, let's take the most logical path to our answer. God loves us, God loves us so much that He gave us his only son to die for all of us, and alls God asked is that we love one another...

Now, Satan hates that people are living long, full lives. People were starting to get along. Satan doesn't want happiness, he wants chaos. Satan causes trauma and malcontent and evil.

Satan longs for life. Satan longs for love. Satan wants people to start hating God, and the best way to do that is to turn God into the bad one. Maybe Satan thinks if he can get enough people to turn on

ROBIN

(Continued)

God, by using God's own love against Him, maybe Satan's glass will start to fill. Ya think?

Therefore, by deduction, AIDS is not a punishment but a jealous child throwing a tantrum because someone else has what it wants...Life.

There.

Satan is behind this. And he's behind all them people who say not to listen to me. They don't want you to confuse their hate.

Does this all make sense? Would you agree with me?

And just to be clear, I ain't all that religious now...maybe there's a God...maybe there ain't. But if...if we need a deity or something like that to blame; wouldn't it make more sense to blame the evil one, rather than the loving one?

Can I get an amen up in here?

(Robin returns to her seat leaving on her blue.)

(Cyc to white. Cast in half light.)

AARON

In 1994, HIV Positive actor Dack Rambo, the guy who played Jack Ewing on the night-time soap "Dallas" died on a Monday at the age of 52.

ROBERT

Randy Shilts, a journalist covering AIDS for the San Francisco chronicle and author of "And The Band Played On: People, Politics and the AIDS Epidemic"

ROBERT

(Continued)

dies from AIDS on February 17, 1994. Shilts announced the previous year that he had been diagnosed with AIDS in 1987. At a time when people died from AIDS within months, Randy Shilts had a seven-year lifespan.

MARION

1995, Greg Louganis admits he is HIV positive. As of 2015, he is still alive.

AARON

Wait. I can top that one. Magic Johnson, big old, heterosexual basketball player, announced he was HIV Positive in 1991...three years earlier. He is still alive in 2015.

HELEN

What is this? A pissing contest? You want to write your name in the snow? Go ahead. But, famous names aside, in 2002 the approximate number of *known* HIV positive people, worldwide, is 22,000,000. Imagine that. 22,000,000 people with HIV, and there still isn't a cure.

MARION

That is a lot.

HELEN

You want to put that number into perspective? 22,000,000 people is larger than the entire population of the continent of Australia.

ROBERT

33,000,000 in 2009.

HELEN

In 2015, one in six people who are living with HIV do not know they carry the virus.

(Jared puts on something purple.)

AARON

And one in four of the new infections reported are heterosexual males between the ages of 14 and 24.

ROBERT

Is there any way to stop it?

HELEN

There has to be.

MARION

The question is: Where do we go from here?

(Cyc to purple. Cast in half light.)

JARED

Really, momma? There's a pot of gold at the end of the rainbow?

HELEN

A pot of gold and a heart of love.

JARED

Where does the gold come from?

HELEN

On top of rainbow clouds, my child. From the top of rainbow clouds.

JARED

Rainbow clouds.

Rainbow clouds are those thin clouds that just hover in the sky. You can't really see them, and then they pass in front of the sun and give it a hazy halo of color. A rainbow halo. A rainbow cloud. But you have to be careful because you can go blind trying to look at one, but they're one of the most beautiful sights above the ground.

If heaven's on a cloud, well, I know it's on a rainbow cloud.

Momma told me there is a pot of gold at the end of every rainbow. A pot of gold. The answer. That's what it is, right?

The answer to everything is at the end of a rainbow.

Rainbows show what beauty can truly be when everything works together. All the colors line up and...boom...a multicolored signature of love. No ugly greed there. Just a hug from the heavens.

I'm not talking about the science of a rainbow. I'm not talking about the theological implications of the great flood. I'm letting you know that a rainbow is love because nature is reminding you that it sometimes washes away the dust...Does some housekeeping.

Rain makes a mess...but then there's a rainbow, helping us to look up to the sky at its beauty, rather than at the muck around our feet. I hate the mud. On my shoes, on my car tires, on the sidewalk.

JARED

(Continued)

Ever notice that? When things are going terrible, we forget all the beauty out there. We concentrate on the mud. When things are going great, we think only of the rainbow, but forget the mud.

When I'm in love, it's the most wonderful feeling in the world. It's great to know you matter to someone.

When I'm alone...my head hangs low, and I see nothing but the grime. I hate being alone. I hate not having someone there to hold my hand.

I'll find love again.

I know it.

I have a crush on my neighbor. He's really cute and wears a revealing swimsuit when he works in his garden.

Yes, I'm gay. I don't like people knowing that about me. It's been my biggest downfall.

My neighbor. My neighbor. He's not married. I think he's gay. I have this fantasy of walking by while he's working on his garden. He stops, looks at me, and we smile. He tells me I look tired, invites me inside where we laugh, drink a little, and then we kiss, and then we...

Blush.

Look! A unicorn!

(The cast looks where he pointed.)

Made you look.

(Cast back to signature poses.)

Why is it that people believe in fantasies?

They need them. Some deep-seeded desire to see the world as beautiful as can be imagined...but that's just it. It's imagined.

JARED

(Continued)

Four years ago, my lover died.

Suicide.

Maybe I'm to blame, maybe I'm not. I haven't figured that one out, yet. He believed in fantasies. He believed if you tried hard enough, anything was possible.

Well, my life didn't become any easier, and his fantasies never became real. He tried, but it was just not meant to be.

Kevin, my lover, partner...he would take me to fantasy places where the world was beautiful and clean. No one knew hatred...They only understood love. Unfortunately, those dreams were just for the two of us relaxing with a glass of wine in front of the fireplace and some mellow music playing in the background.

I loved our date nights. I loved watching the moon slowly gliding across the sky, the stars blink-el-ing and twink-el-ing.

If we stayed up late enough, we would watch the sun slowly rise over the horizon. God, that was fascinating. The warmth it radiated brought forth the smell of...of...clean flowers, of nature doing its work. Of life.

Patience was rewarded by watching the Morning Glories slowly awaken into a profusion of harmonious color.

I would lay there long after Kevin had fallen asleep and watch his chest rise and fall. I often wondered what he was dreaming about.

I loved him.

He loved me.

JARED

(Continued)

We were perfect together.

I would lay my head on his chest and listen to his gentle heartbeat...a heartbeat that he promised beat only for me...that heartbeat would lull me to sleep.

I had safety. Security. He was there...for me. I would ask God to never let it end, but it had to. Nothing is forever. Nothing.

Sometimes it's hard to see beauty...but I try. It's hard to allow myself that pleasure. After Kevin committed suicide, part of me died, too. I couldn't open up and allow myself to love anyone. I needed seclusion. Sometimes, I still need it.

I needed to forgive him for making me hate him. I had to forgive myself for hating him...hating me. Maybe I was the one who killed...forgive and move forward. Forgive and move forward.

After my grief subsided, I went a little wild. I needed to find another Kevin. I needed that security. I fucked around a lot, but that's not the way to form lasting relationships, everyone just thinks you're a slut, and I'm not that...Self-denial...I was a *slut*! I just couldn't face myself with that fact. I guess I hoped if people saw me sleeping around, someone would come to my rescue. But all it did was leave me empty...emptier and lonelier than I was before.

Is it possible to go back to the way things were?

I did meet this new guy, Mark. He was a close runner-up to Kevin.

Mark was more realistic. He took things at face value and left them at that...I could never replace Kevin, but Mark was a great substitute.

JARED

(Continued)

Mark had only one flaw...He loved strange meat. Oh, for those of you who don't speak the lingo, it means he liked to sleep around.

I don't think he would have ever hurt me, but he did.

You see, Mark believed in fun first. Not safety. As much as I loved him, he caught the virus...the disease.

(Slowly...First time we hear the words)

Acquired Immune Deficiency Syndrome.

ROBERT

AIDS.

JARED

AIDS.

He wanted to live, but it's hard to keep fighting when you know it's a losing battle. Everyone dies from this. Everyone. No one can beat it. Dammit, look what trouble you got us into. No one can beat AIDS. No one.

AARON

He was a man.

MARION

Men are supposed to be able to conquer the world.

JARED

He tried to live. He didn't want to leave me. He didn't.

But he knew he had to...

JARED
(Continued)

He was in and out of the hospital so much...Our friends stopped coming by, his family rejected him, even his sister, who promised she'd be with him until the end, stopped visiting.

I didn't turn my back on Mark. I stayed with him. Every day, dressing up in that damn biohazard suit. Every day, holding his hand through latex gloves. Every day, praying for a miracle.

He was in a coma just before the end. At least he went...peacefully. Yeah. Like knowing that helped me a lot. I couldn't bear to see another person I loved dying in pain. Agonizing pain.

But, before he died, Mark lived in that pain. His skin breaking out into a wild, itchy rash. His mouth became more and more dehydrated until his teeth dropped out. His long, beautiful blond hair fell out in handfuls. He slowly withered away in front of my very eyes.

I was at his bedside when he went into his coma. When no one was looking, I took off that stupid glove, and held his hand. His hand was cold, but soft. I could feel his pulse. He tried hard to squeeze my hand back, but he was too weak. I lifted his hand to my lips and kissed it under that awful mask. My eyes never left his. Never. I saw them fill with tears, and, in that raspy voice of his, he said,

ROBERT

"I love you."
(Pause)
"I love you."

JARED

I told him I loved him, too.

ROBERT

"Stay with me. Let me rest."

JARED

I felt his hand fall limp. His beautiful...oh so beautiful...eyes closed for the last time...and...

I couldn't see straight. I wanted to die. I had to. There was something wrong with me. In four years I had killed to lovers. What was wrong with my blood...

(Quickly)

my love! Why wasn't it strong enough to keep people from dying? Why does everything have to end? I just wanted one more day with him well. I wanted to hold him, and treat him like Kevin...

(Quickly)

Mark! To say I'm sorry, dammit. I'm sorry. I can't keep this damn thing from killing you.

Don't leave me. Don't leave me.

Why in the hell couldn't I have one more day?

Are you listening to me, God? Just one day. You could've let enough things go by without having to take my lover.

Why?

Why me?

Why did you allow such a thing as AIDS to come into our lives? Are we that bad?

(Soft)

Are we?

(Composes self)

JARED

(Continued)

When *they* decided to pull the plug on his life support. I had a glimmer of hope. His heart...his heart kept beating for me. He still loved me...and then...

(Uses finger to simulate lifeline in air)

Three...heart...beats...

(Finger simulates flat line as ALL, except Jared release a 'last-sigh'. Jared's finger stops and one point and does not move.)

I wanted to put my head on his chest and hear them...

(Finger down - Soft voice.)

But those bastards wouldn't let me touch him. Why not? It was impossible to catch his AIDS that way. No one should die alone when there are others willing to hold them.

Why can't I touch him?

Why can't I hold his hand?

(Pause)

Why did he have to die?

I don't want gold on top of those clouds. No. No. I want Kevin and Mark waiting for me. I want to look up and see their hands reaching for me, touching me...pulling me up to them.

That's my fantasy!

The pot of gold is at the end of the rainbow, but it keeps getting further and further away. The gold is from the top of rainbow clouds, but you can't see it because you'll go blind. I need to see them. I need to hold them. Why is everything I want just out of my reach?

I need them.

JARED
(Continued)
I need their friendship.
   I need a friend.

ALL
(Standing)
I'll be your friend.

JARED
Just one friend, that's all I need.

ALL
(Takes one step toward Jared. Cast will
remain in shadow and come toward the
light)
I'll be your friend.

JARED
Forever?

ALL
(Takes one step toward Jared)
Forever.

JARED
No matter what?

ALL
(Takes one step toward Jared)
No matter what.

JARED

(Pause)
I have AIDS.

> (Everyone, except Aaron, turns, military
> fashion, and return to their seats, and ease
> into their signature poses.)

AARON

I'll be your friend.

JARED

That's all I need.

AARON

One friend.

JARED

You'll stay by me? Hold my hand? Let me look into
your eyes as I die?

AARON

You're not going to die.

JARED

Do you promise that your eyes will be the eyes I look
into when I leave this planet?

(Pause)

AARON

I swear.

JARED

(Hugs Aaron)
Don't leave me.

AARON

Never. You're my friend.

(Jared will release his hold on Aaron and
slowly walk back to his chair to assume the
position he held prior to the beginning of the
monologues. As Jared crosses; each cast
member will slowly stand into position they
held prior to the beginning of the
monologues. They say the following lines,
ethereal in nature, as they stand. As they
stand, fantasy lighting begins to transition to
normal stage lighting.)

HELEN

They'll last. They've learned.

MARION

She'll never die.

ROBERT

My baby brother.

AARON

Leave the children alone.

ROBIN

Blame the bad one, instead of the good one.

                    JARED
Where do we go from here?

          (All are in place. Fantasy lighting out,
          normal stage lights up.)

                    ALL
He has what?

                    JARED
Brent found out he has AIDS.

                    ROBERT
That sucks.

                    HELEN
You think he'll be okay?

                    JARED
He has a long haul in front of him...

          (The pace builds from this point to Marion's
          'explosion')

                    MARION
That's what happens to fags. Fuck. AIDS. Die.

                    HELEN
You don't have to be gay to get it, Marion.

                    ROBERT
And sex isn't the only way.

MARION
Men are rats. Rats bring plagues.

AARON
Women get it.

MARION
Gay men get it.

HELEN
Ralph's gay, and he doesn't have it.

MARION
Men are disease. Parasites. Men are hateful, vile
insects that we need to be drawn and quartered. If it
weren't for men, there'd be no disease.

AARON
You're so screwed in the head, it's amazing!

MARION
Fuck you!

JARED
Fuck you! What would you say if I told you I had
AIDS?

MARION
            (Explodes)
That you deserve it.

            (Everyone stops in disbelief.)

STAGE MANAGER
(Off, or can appear on stage in harried state)
What is wrong with you people? I said, "Places!"
Dammit! This show is going on with or without you.

(Helen squares her shoulders and locks her arm into Aaron's as they exit. Robin exits behind Robert. Marion and Jared stare at each other for a moment...Jared grabs a serving tray and faces audience.)

JARED
(English accent - respectful)
Your light is calling, mum.

(Marion and Jared stand in tableau as the lights fade to...)

BLACKOUT

END ACT ONE

Fallen Guardian Angels

Act Two

Setting: The setting is the same as Act One. The tea cart is center stage.

At Rise: The stage is empty. Aaron enters and will begin to loosen his tie, but notices the paper Jared tossed aside from Act One. He picks it up and is about to toss it in the wastepaper basket when he stops, will smooth it out, and reads. He starts to fold the paper when Helen and Robert enter. Aaron will put the paper in his pocket.

A note for this act: There are no exits after the main entrance. Actors who are on stage but not utilized during a 'fantasy' scene should freeze into position and basically become props on stage.

AARON
You think we have a hit?

ROBERT
I'd say we have a hit.

(Marion and Robin enter.)

HELEN
I think we have a reason to celebrate.

ROBIN
Did you see all the people standing?

AARON
Where's Jared?

ROBIN
He was talking to Ralph.

HELEN
My Ralph?

ROBIN
Yeah. All secretive. Bet they're planning on throwing you a party.

HELEN
Sure.

ROBERT
(Crossing to Marion)
Good show, Dyke-zilla.

MARION
(Distant)
You, too.

ROBERT
No bitchy comeback? Are you okay?

MARION
Fine. Just a lot on my mind.

(Jared enters. The rest stop and stare. He realizes everyone is looking at him.)

JARED
That was fun. I'm glad I decided to do it.

HELEN

Yes. Me, too. Ralph told me I should try theatre. So much energy. Two shows under my belt.

AARON

It always helps me cope with outside life. It's a great way to forget the rest of the world. I needed this break.

ROBERT

I haven't seen you at many auditions lately...

AARON

Three years. Not since Tricia died.

ROBERT

Sorry.

AARON

Don't be. It's time I rejoin the living. You know? Tricia and I met doing a show together. She was with me on stage tonight.

JARED

I love theatre, but there are so many superstitions...I mean, they're great, but ghosts and bards and all that. Like when you all made me go outside and turn around three times and spit because I said...um...the name of that show that we're not supposed to say.

HELEN

I think we all do it our first time. I wish I had started doing shows earlier, though. Now all I get to be is matrons, mothers and maids.

ROBIN

I started doing shows in high school, but I stopped after I graduated. Just a show here and there when...well, like Aaron said...When I needed a break from reality, to give me a chance to be someone else. And my brother always loves me in shows. I did this one for him.

HELEN

(To Marion)
Why do you do theatre?

ROBERT

Community service.

MARION

Screw you...I did this one for Nicole. It's her favorite show.

JARED

I thought opening nights would last forever.

AARON

Never do. Just seem like it.

ROBERT

We're all here! Who gets the "Fickle Finger" award for tonight?

HELEN

The what?

ROBIN

There's a tradition at this theatre. The worst screw up of the night gets a little award. Someone made it on opening night of the first show done here. Every show after that, the award circulates to the cast member causing the biggest mistake of the night.

AARON

It's sort of a way to try to keep everyone from messing up.

ROBIN

Right. But the person who gets it on closing night is supposed to get cast in the next show.

HELEN

Oh! Sort of like the woman who catches a bouquet at a wedding.

AARON

Exactly.

JARED

Who gets it tonight?

AARON
                (Grabs award from table - hands it to
                Jared during...)
You do. For the best screw up of the night.

JARED

Me?

HELEN

Jared messed up?

ROBERT

Big time. You weren't on stage yet, but the line is supposed to go...
(English Accent)
"Pardon me, Mr. Newberg, but Mr. Albus is dingalinging you about playing soccer."

AARON

And genius here says...
(English Accent)
"Soccer, sir, Mr. Albus is playing with your dingaling."

(All chuckle)

HELEN

Thank goodness we're doing a comedy.

JARED

(Holding up "award")
I would like to thank the Academy...
   Great, now I'm stuck with this damn thing.

AARON

Don't worry, you'll give it to someone.

ROBIN

Plenty of time for you to give it to someone else.

HELEN
Congratulations, honey!
                (Indicates Wine Glasses)
Anyone up for some celebrating?

JARED
I'll take a little, but I'm driving...so not too much.

ROBERT
After the opening night performance, the actors usually sit for a bit and talk...It'll have time to go through your system.

JARED
It all seems like a dream.

AARON
                (Aaron will say the following lines as he
                pours. As the 'wine' (water) leaves the carafe
                and fills the glass, the liquid will become
                each person's signature color...Red, Orange,
                etc.)
Theatre is a dream. It's a fantasy. What happens on stage is not real, but the reflection of how life was at the time. When we watch live actors on stage, whatever the play, whatever the situation, we are watching history. The lines they speak could have been written two weeks ago, or hundreds of years ago...We watch history come to life as we watch Romeo woo Juliet, or Elwood speak to an invisible rabbit.

AARON
(Continued: All glasses poured.)
So, my friend, enjoy the illusion, enjoy the
fantasy...for, after we walk out of the theatre; time
catches up, and we are back in reality.

JARED
I like fantasy. I like wishes....
(Takes his glass)
If I could have one fantasy...It would be a cure for
the world.

AARON
(Takes his glass)
There are no problems that humankind couldn't
overcome.

HELEN
(Takes her glass)
If we all work together.

ROBERT
(Takes his glass)
And put our differences aside.

ROBIN
(Takes her glass)
Amen.

MARION
(Takes her glass)
Salud!

(They all raise their glasses, and take a sip. Marion goes back to her chair with her glass)

ROBERT

May tomorrow be a better day.

(Cyc to white)

ROBIN

(Grabs roses)
Time to hand out the roses! Yay!

HELEN

We get roses, too?

ROBERT

It's not like they pay us.

(Robin will distribute one rose to each person.)

ROBIN

(Handing Jared the white rose.)
For the theatre virgin...

HELEN

(Pulling Marion aside.)
Marion? Are you okay?

MARION

Nicole's cancer is bad. She was asleep before I came to the theatre. I wish she could've been here tonight.

HELEN

I'm sure she's thinking about you...

(Cyc to Green)

MARION

You don't understand...She is my inspiration, my indecision, my indiscretion. I live my life to have our passions deeply incensed. While I kiss her lips, fervent lusts escape my brain and burst from my shaking groin...matching grinds from her wet pleasure, wanting time to encase skin within the envelope of her hot fold of declamation. I welcome her treaty of slow death, yet I spurn her, awaiting the far time when we meet in another life to make love forever in total, insatiable, eternity. It is this love that keeps me alive.

HELEN

Such a love so deep will never go unrewarded. Keep your hopes up and dreams high. Many people have beaten cancer, Marion. Many. That's the God's honest truth.

(Cyc to white)

(This must be done quickly: Helen will move the tea-cart off to one side while Robert and Robin grab the two trunks on either side of the stage, bring them center and sit them on a slight diagonal, at this point, the trunks will become a bench. Aaron and Jared sit on the bench for the next few lines.)

AARON
I finally asked that girl out that we saw last week.

JARED
Cool.

AARON
It was awesome. She and I hit it off so well...and, you know, she agrees to go back to my place for a little.... hokey-pokey.

JARED
I hope you had safe sex.

AARON
Of course, I had a condom on, but she wanted to make sure she didn't get pregnant or sick, so she went to the bathroom and got her paraphernalia. We were getting into it, and I was having a great time, but then I found out she was using spermicidal foam...by the time I realized this, I looked like a rabid dog.

JARED
Oh...god....dude.

(Marion picks up the phone and dials)

ROBIN
(To Helen)
What's up with her?

                              HELEN
Her partner has cancer. Not doing too good. She's
worried.

                              MARION
          (Into phone)
Three, east, please...

          (Marion will ignore others)

                              ROBERT
Three, east? That's the AIDS ward.

                              AARON
It could be a different hospital.

                              HELEN
Ralph and Gary volunteer there through that
Whoopie group.

                              ROBIN
Whoopie?

                              HELEN
Something like "Helping People With AIDS".

                              ROBERT
Oh...Whappa...They're a group that goes to the
AIDS ward, talk with people who have the
disease...They're there for them when...
          (Trails off)

                              AARON
When they die.

HELEN

Yes. It's a hard group to be a part of. I mean, meeting someone and having them leave you within a few weeks. But, still, having someone to communicate with, to talk to...

JARED

Sometimes they can't talk. Sometimes they're in a coma.

HELEN

It's having someone there that matters, Jared.

JARED

I know.

ROBIN

How do you know about Whappa, Robert?

ROBERT

They help my friend, Vincent. He's not doing good.

ROBIN

Why we even talking about the AIDS ward?
          (To Helen)
I thought you said it was cancer.

HELEN

That's what Marion told me.

ROBIN

We all have two sides. Maybe she doesn't know.

JARED

Doesn't know that Three-East is the AIDS ward? You have to wear all that crap to get in there.

(Realizes he may be saying too much)

She might be a man-hating bitch, but she's not stupid.

ROBIN

Everyone is capable of lying...Or hiding the truth. It's being able to face yourself in the mirror that matters. But, even then, we can be deceptive. If you look at yourself in the mirror, is that the true you, or is it the opposite of you?

(Cyc to Blue)

JARED

It is the true you.

ROBIN

No, it's not. It's reversed.

HELEN

The opposite of who you are.

ROBERT

Remember that exercise the director had us do? If you raise your right hand in the mirror, the reflection raises its left.

ROBIN

Right. And just like the mirror, what we show others is what we want to see. Sometimes, that deception is so deep that we see the reflection of what we want to be, but not who we truly are.

AARON

You can't hide the truth by refracting a reflection.

ROBIN

No, but you can hide the reflection by twisting the mirror.

Think about it. The truth is only as real as the person telling it to you. There are always the different truths we hear. What did we first hear about AIDS? That is was GRIDS...a Gay Related Immune Deficiency, and people took that to be the truth. Only gay people get it. The news twisted the truth, and people believed it.

Then they started calling it AIDS, and said everyone could get it, but some people cling to the first truth, even though it is no longer valid. To them, it is their truth.

They held up the mirror to the disease and made it appear to be what they wanted it to be...a way of supporting their own hatred and bigotry. There are women out there with the disease, straight men, from all walks of life..

We need to break that mirror and make sure the real truth gets out there.

(Marion hangs up phone and joins group)

JARED

But if there are so many different versions out there,
how do we know which one is real?

ROBERT

We learn.

AARON

Get in touch with reality.

ROBIN

Find out the truth about things.

ROBERT

But isn't the truth the hardest thing to find?

ROBIN

Not to find...no, not that...it's...it's...

MARION

It's the hardest to accept.

ROBERT

So how do we avoid fear?

AARON

Knowledge.

ROBERT

And how do we avoid bigotry?

ROBIN

Understanding.

ROBERT

Sex?

JARED

What?

ROBERT

Everyone is afraid of sex, right?

HELEN

Oh, honey, it's been so long since I've had sex I forget who plays with the chicken.
>   (Closest cast member leans in and whispers
>   to Helen)

Cock....
>   (Quick Pause)

Cock?

ROBERT

Um...Okay...Everyone is afraid of sex, but what would make sex more enjoyable?

AARON

A partner.

ROBERT

Be serious.

JARED

You think I'm not?
     Fine. Fine...I think it's time everyone embraces celibacy.

ROBIN

What you smoking, baby? Puff, puff, pass...

ROBERT

Why do people insist that AIDS means celibacy? No sex? There is nothing wrong with two consenting adults sharing intimate moments...Gay, straight, lesbian...We are now in what people call the 'sexual revolution' and we want to take steps backwards? Why can't we encourage safe-sex? Condoms, frottage...

JARED

No glove no love?

ROBERT

Right.

JARED

Get the same satisfaction from a blow-up doll.

MARION

Just gather up the men with AIDS and put them in their own community.

ROBERT

Like an AIDS camp?
   Putting people in camps because they're different. Correct me if I'm wrong...but wasn't that Hitler's idea?

MARION

Maybe...but a lot of people think that we should.

ROBERT
A lot of Nazis thought that, too.

MARION
Then ship them off to some faraway island with disco balls and white foam all over the place. They'll be happy.

JARED
Welcome to Homoslavia...

MARION
Exactly...The best way to avoid a problem is to contain the problem.

ROBERT
So AIDS victims are a problem?

MARION
For damn sure.

ROBERT
Is there any compassion in your heart?

MARION
Look, Robert...I say what I feel. AIDS victims are nothing but a burden on society, taking up space until they die...wasting taxpayer money for hospital beds, medicines, medical staff. Face the truth, gay-boy, if fags were kept away from the rest of us, none

MARION
(Continued)
of this would've ever happened. They did it to themselves. Why should I pay for it? They should just die and stop wasting space.

JARED
They are not a waste of space. It's people like you, who hate them for doing nothing wrong, that's the waste.

MARION
AIDS is here because faggots can't keep their little tower of death to themselves. They should hold up and wait to die.

ROBERT
Is that what we do? Shun them? You really want to live in that sort of society?

MARION
It's how I feel. If that's not where we're headed, then where do we go from here?

(Cyc transitions from yellow to purple)

JARED
You know what I saw tonight? While we were taking our bows? I saw a guy with Kaposi Sarcoma lesions on his forehead.
(Indicates)
Right here. Did anyone else see him?
(No. Robin tense.)

JARED

(Continued)

I did. He was sitting in the third row with someone...When I saw him smiling at us, I couldn't help but wink at him from the line up.

I know what those lesions mean. I know he has AIDS.

But I looked at the audience, and they weren't looking at him, they were looking at us, and that guy was happy. He was someplace where no one cared about his condition. Never mind that most of them probably didn't know what it is...He was treated like a human, and isn't that what we all are?

Human?

He was not a waste of space.

MARION

If I saw him, I would know he was a slutty fag.

ROBIN

Take a pill, Marion. That man Jared's talking about is no slutty fag.

MARION

Like you know.

ROBIN

That was my brother, and if you call him a slutty fag one more time, we'll need your understudy tomorrow night.

HELEN

We have understudies?

ROBIN

My brother is straight and a virgin, Marion. The lady who rammed her car into his was a drunk-ass bitch who was too busy trying to find "Wake Me Up Before You Go Go" on the radio to pay attention to the road.

MARION

You can't get AIDS from a car accident.

ROBIN

He needed surgery and blood...something like five pints...I don't know, but he was hurt. He got AIDS from a transfusion.

MARION

They process that blood.

ROBIN

One out of every hundred bags...Learn this shit. You think they want to spend money testing every donor?

MARION

Your brother must have had some gay in him. AIDS only finds gay people.

ROBIN

You're sounding like my pops. "Women don't get it." "Gays get it." My brother says he is straight, but my dad won't even listen.
        (Imitates 'dad')
"Must be a flower." "Must be a poofer"
        (Normal)

ROBIN

(Continued)
That's all my pops says anymore.

MARION

Your dad knows his shit.

ROBIN

Brian is not gay, Marion.

MARION

Then it must be for men.
(Pause)
Everything we hear says women won't get it.

HELEN

We haven't heard everything.

AARON

They told us AIDS was a possibility when Tricia
needed blood.
(Pause)
They made us sign a waiver. I don't know why. It
wasn't like...It wouldn't make a difference.

(Cyc transitions to Red)

MARION

Wait...Tricia? Your wife?

AARON

When we found out she had AIDS, all we could
think was that she would break it, she would defeat
it, she was the one who would win. We were wrong.

MARION

She was a woman.

AARON

And she had AIDS.

MARION

How...I mean...How?

AARON

Needle.

JARED

I.V. drugs? But I thought you said she died in delivery.

AARON

I know what you I told you, Jared. I know I lied...

JARED

Is that why I see you at Mercy?

ROBERT

You were holding a baby. He's about six months old.

AARON

My son. He's almost three. AIDS has caused a sort of developmental inertia. He still has the body of a four week old.

MARION

He's only three? Then he can't have AIDS.

AARON

There was a less than eight percent chance he'd get it, Marion. Less than eight percent. Tricia followed all the doctor's orders. She didn't breastfeed. She was terrified to hold him...sometimes she was too weak to hold him.

(Robert hands Aaron the 'baby' from act one)
On those days, I would hold him up for her. One time, she allowed Shawn to grab her finger while I held him. She looked at him and said she was sorry. And then she sang that song...

ROBIN

(Sings softly under Aaron's lines - "All Through The Night")
Sleep my child, and peace attend thee. All through the night. Guardian angels God will send thee. All through the night.

AARON

...and Shawn smiled. He knew his mom. He knew that they held each other. We knew that he forgave her.

Everyone asks me if she went peacefully. I wasn't there.

I didn't get the Hollywood ending. I didn't get the life-long last moment that I can cling to every time something goes wrong and I need her. I was at work. A Friday.

Tricia died alone.

(Helen will put on a red surgeon's mask and cap)
Oh, God, I wasn't there for her.

AARON

(Continued)

When I held Shawn after his mother died; I took off the glove and let him hold my finger. It was the *first time* our skin had ever met. I wasn't allowed to touch him because of his AIDS. I wasn't allowed to kiss his forehead, his cheek...

HELEN

(Nurse: Mask should not cover her mouth)

You need to wear your gloves.

AARON

Excuse me?

HELEN

Gloves. We have rules to help protect your health.

AARON

He's my son.

HELEN

He has AIDS.

AARON

I know he has AIDS. I'm standing in the middle of the AIDS ward surrounded by people telling me to be careful. People who are supposed to be helping these patients, but are afraid to touch them.

He should be at home, with me...learning his alphabet...getting into mischief.

HELEN

Sir, put on your gloves or I will ban you from this ward...

AARON

(Hands Marion the baby)
Ban me?
(At Helen)
Ban me? Shawn's my son. I'm his father. You are not banning me from seeing him.

HELEN

Sir, you need to wear protection...

AARON

Protection? From my son?

HELEN

We have rules for this ward...

AARON

Let me tell you about rules, lady. First, there is no rule against me holding my son. You cannot stop me. Second, my rule is if you even think about banning me from seeing my son, I will ruin your life.

HELEN

That's a little extreme, sir. We're only thinking about your health.

AARON

Nothing out there says that any of this crap works. Your little mask...your biohazard suit...your cold hearts. AIDS is not airborne.

HELEN
That has not been determined.

AARON
If it was, your hospital wouldn't have these people here. You cannot catch AIDS from the air. You cannot catch AIDS from drinking out of the same cup. The only way you can catch AIDS from a toilet seat is if you sit down before the other guy gets up.

Stop punishing the people with the disease. They did nothing wrong.

My son did nothing wrong.

I did nothing wrong.

HELEN
But he has AIDS.

(Helen removes all traces of red and returns to her beginning point)

MARION
He's just a baby.

AARON
And he has AIDS, Marion. He isn't gay. He isn't straight.

He is love.

ROBERT
People need to accept that AIDS has no boundaries. It gets into who it can and kills them. Stop trying to find scapegoats. If we spent as much energy trying

ROBERT

(Continued)

to find a cure as we did trying to place blame, AIDS would already be a memory.

(Robert and Marion will unfold the blanket and use it to cover the bench that sits center. The bench will now become a casket. It is now the 'elephant in the room' that will go unnoticed until needed. Robin will cross to Aaron and hand him her rose.)

JARED

But where do we go from here?

AARON

(Kneels for a moment at the casket. A moment of reflection before he places two roses on the casket. Stands.)

I wish I knew.

HELEN

I'm sure there are scientists and doctors working around the clock trying to find a cure.

JARED

The cure is out there, sitting at the end of a rainbow.

HELEN

That's it...be positive.

JARED

The closer you get to the rainbow...the further it moves away...That's the problem...Science trumps beauty.

ROBERT

Not always.

I can see it in your eyes. The prism effect only works when you are far away from it. You can never reach the end of the rainbow because it's actually an illusion.

Fuck that. Throw away your science for a moment. Stop trying to analyze beauty.

At what age did you stop believing in Santa Claus? The Easter Bunny?

The year your brain brought science into the picture, and you realized these things could not be real...They were unscientific.

But those were the moments of hope. Going to sleep on Christmas eve, believing you were a good boy or girl, and knowing Santa would bring you a shitload of toys.

I miss my childhood.

I miss innocent wonder.

Why did we have to grow up?

JARED

I want to believe. I want to have hope.

AARON

At least you get a chance to know hope....I never had that wonder. I got a dreidel and some chocolate coins. That's the only time I hated being Jewish...I

AARON
(Continued)
wanted a tree and a fat philanthropist flying down my chimney.

JARED
I want researchers to find a way to beat AIDS. I want a cure.

AARON
(His own little world)
I wanted toys. I got socks. You know how excited it is to get over socks? Ooh, they're black and they fit. Wow. Hold me back.

Show 'em off at school, you say? Definitely.

Oh? You got a Ranger Rick picnic set and a new bicycle?
(Lifts up pant leg to model his socks)
Check these babies out. From the K-Mart collection. And I got five more pairs just like 'em.

(Pause)

ROBERT
They will stop AIDS one day, Jared. Wait and see.

MARION
There's no way to stop AIDS. Once it's out there, it finds some guy and gets into him. Gloves, rubbers, all that crap...Nothing can stop it. It just gets into any man it can and kills.

JARED
And here comes our little ray of sunshine...

HELEN

It's scary. I mean, she's right. AIDS kills.

I love Ralph and Gary so much, but sometimes I find myself worrying not "if" they'll get AIDS, but "when".

You know what the C.D.C. says? That one out of every six people in America will have AIDS by 1990. One in six.

ROBIN

Disturbing. It's scary...I mean, what if I'm next?

ROBERT

You can't think like that. Paranoia isn't the answer.

ROBIN

We can't? A lot of people are scared. When you don't know what's going on, or how to stop something...Ya know?

ROBERT

Okay. So, everyone is afraid of AIDS, but no one really knows anything about it. We have to learn the truth about AIDS, and then accept that truth.

How does AIDS get into a person's body and eventually kill them?

HELEN

It enters the body through blood-borne pathogens or other bodily fluids. It's an opportunistic virus that attacks your immune system, leaving it damaged and unable to fight viruses and diseases. One millionth our size, and it renders a person helpless.

AARON

Wow. And, for those of us who aren't med students?

MARION

Everyone's taken courses in microbiology, right?

JARED

Sure...and my dentist isn't a sadist.

HELEN

I wish there was an easier way to communicate this.

ROBERT

Well, as to what I understand...AIDS is a...a...
dinosaur.

(Cyc to yellow)

ROBIN

A what?

ROBERT

I like to watch reruns of the "Flintstones". They
have cute, adorable Dino. We have the big, scary,
Try-Anything-Once Rex...Follow me? Okay, our red
blood cells are the cavemen, doing cavemanny type
things: taking out the garbage, fixing the microwave
oven, sacrificing virgins to the volcano god.

AARON

A virgin? That's a terrible thing to waste.

ROBERT

Those cavemen are out doing their thing...protecting their environment, gathering food, doing what needs to be done to sustain the community.

But there are dangers out there...so the cavemen have a group of Pitbull-asaurs...They didn't have to do anything to get them, either. The cavemen have had these pitbull-asaurs since their conception.

MARION

No puns intended.

ROBERT

The pitbull-asaurs represent our white blood cells that fend off diseases. They protect the cavemen from dinosaurs and poison ivy.

JARED

I don't get it.

ROBERT

Okay. Our bodies are the community. The cavemen are our red blood cells, carrying out their daily routine of keeping the community, our body, healthy, and the pitbull-asaurs are our white blood cells...those are the cells that fight off the common cold, the flu, or any sort of something-something that isn't right in the body.

Got it?

JARED

Cool.

ROBERT
Are you a caveman, or a pitbull-asaur?

JARED
(Pause - Becomes a caveman)
Get firewood, I'll warm up the car.

ROBERT
So, a caveman?

JARED
("Normal")
It's hard to act like a dog that wants to eat viruses.
So, yeah, I'm a caver.

AARON
(Caveman)
I just invented this round thing. I think I'll call it a
wheel.

ROBIN
(Disgusted)
Call it a pizza. I'm starving.

HELEN
Has anyone seen the newspaper?

JARED
Don't be silly, we're cavemen. Cavemen don't read.

HELEN
Then has anyone seen the phone?

> (The entire cast does a quick three count to look at the 'phone person' the Stage Manager pointed out in the first act, and then back into the action)

ROBERT

Hush!

Okay, so we've established it. The cavemen are the immune system of the first person.

But no one likes to be alone, and our first community   soon   meets   another community...another person...

> (Marion and Helen pair up. Robin, who seems disinterested, agrees to be part of the second 'group')

...and they find the second community neato.

AARON

Neato?

ROBIN

An archaic term from which the slang "tight" derived.

AARON

Word.

MARION

Back to Robert.

ROBERT

Thank you.

The first community finds the second community tight.

ROBIN

Better.

JARED

Um....never mind.

ROBERT

We'll call the second community "John."

MARION

Great pun.

HELEN

I don't get it.

MARION

"John", you know...Like a one-night-stand.

HELEN
        (Rubs watch)
Lay off the John jokes.

JARED

Why do they call them "One-Night-Stands" when everyone is on their backs?

ROBIN

Will you all shut up?

ROBERT

Thank you, Robin.
   Well, John doesn't realize they carry with them the egg that holds the

ROBERT
(Continued: Ominous 'singing')
Da-da-duhh...
(Holds up a plastic purple egg)
Tryanythingonce Rex...
They have one of these eggs in an incubator. Some
community from the past gave it to them, not that
they wanted it, but it's there. I mean, it'll be
explained. They're good people, it's just that...
Nevermind...wait.

JARED
Okay, so the cavers are our blood, the pitbullasaurs
are white blood cells, and the egg is AIDS, right?

ROBERT
Right.

JARED
Cool.

ROBERT
One night, both communities decide to do a ritual
rain-dance.
(The other actors now go into a 'dance' pose
to circle around Robert - they start dancing -
One group clockwise, the other group
counter-clockwise. During the 'dance', Jared
will sneak the purple egg into his possession)
This dance is usually safe to do, as long as the
communities remember to put a special ritual
rubber sheet between them. This is for protection.
Something like...I don't know...a condom perhaps?

AARON

Of course.

ROBERT

Placing the rubber sheet between them is important and easy to do, but the communities decide they don't need it. They're going to settle down and share the crops, so they decide not to use the sheet.
        (Cast stops dancing)
Well, during the dance, the egg...
        (Jared holds up egg)
...splits in half...
        (Jared splits egg)
...and one of the halves washes down the stream...

JARED
        (As he simulates the egg washing down a river)
In the blood or seminal fluids...

ROBERT

...and ends up in the other community's cave. It gets lodged into a small crevice...

MARION
        (Jared plops half of the egg into Marion's bra)
Small? Really?

ROBERT

A crevice of undetermined size...Lodged in there real good where no one notices it.

ROBERT
(Continued)
This is how it happened last time, and how it will continue to do so for many years to come unless we find a way to squash that egg.

And all this took place so quickly...That egg was lost between lighting that celebratory cigarette and promising to exchange cave-numbers.

Hell, they knew they wouldn't need that rubber sheet. This time it was for real.

JARED
And they live happily ever after?

HELEN
A quick relationship like that? No courting, no woo'ing, no moonlight kisses upon a gentle lake while the...

AARON
(Interrupting)
There she goes again...

MARION
(Loud)
A relationship like that, Jared? Get real!

ROBERT
Exactly. A couple of months later, John leaves....No reason.

HELEN
I guess those lines of communication were shut down. Communication is the key to all

HELEN

(Continued)

relationships. Gay. Straight...The day my water broke...

ALL

(Interrupting)

Helen.

ROBERT

Anyway, our first community is in turmoil. They need to find the right clothes so they can find another happening group.

But they still have that egg.

The egg stays hidden for months. No one ever figures it's there.

(Marion will squat down in front of Robert)

Then, it hatches...

MARION

(Being "born". Does a "Jazz Hands" move)

Ta-da!

ROBERT

A tiny, little Tryanythingonce Rex is born. But it doesn't stay tiny for long. That sucker grows like a mother.

(Marion 'matures' into 'dinosaur' and does the "guns" pose)

And it rears its ugly head and attacks the community.

ROBIN

The cavers throw a major freak-out, right?

AARON

And the Pitbullasaurs attack the Rex.

JARED

They're no match.

ROBERT

The Rex chomps those Pits to pieces.

HELEN

Oh, yummers.

(Marion "kills" Helen)

ROBERT

The cavers try everything to kill the Rex.
   They give it yogurt.

JARED

Someone said the bacteria in yogurt kills it.

ROBERT

Doesn't work.
      (Marion "kills" Jared)
   They try to convince the Rex that it isn't alive.

ROBIN

Holistic health...peace and harmony...That'll work!

ROBERT

It doesn't believe them.
      (Marion "kills" Robin)

ROBERT
(Continued)
They even heard of a gimmick that protects the cavers from getting a Rex...

AARON
A condom, perhaps?

ROBERT
...But it's already there.
(Marion "kills" Aaron)
The Rex just grows and grows. Even the new Pitbullasaurs that are in training for the new Rex aren't strong enough. Rex gets stronger while the community grows weaker.

Finally, Rex eats all the cavers.
(Marion lets out a huge belch)
There aren't anymore.

Rex sees this, takes a final bow, and takes what it can to that great Dino-land in the sky.

(Marion 'flies' off to her seat and sits)

HELEN
The end.

ROBERT
Not yet. You see, the community was good at doing the rain-dance, and it did it with several other communities before it died out. Most of the time, they used the ritual rubber sheet, but, every once in a while, they felt they didn't need it, and during those times, another egg made it to another community.

ROBERT
(Continued)

So there are a lot of communities out there with an egg, and most don't even know it. It could take days, weeks, or even months, but, someday, that egg is going to hatch into a mean, huge Tryanythingonce Rex.

ROBIN

Cute story.

HELEN

I like it.

ROBERT

But the moral of the story is?
(Pause)
Use your rubber sheet...no matter how safe the other cavers look!

JARED

I wish everyone would learn that.

ROBIN

Amen.

HELEN

So now we know how it does what it does, but where do we go from here?

(Robert crosses to the casket with his red rose. Kneels and puts rose on casket.)

                              ROBERT
I wish I knew.

          (Cyc to white)

          (Jared stands off to the side, looking
          depressed. Aaron crosses to him.)

                              AARON
Jared? You okay?

                              JARED
I'm fine. Just thoughts going through my head.

                              AARON
What thoughts?

                              JARED
Nothing. The dinosaur. I love dinosaurs.
          (Smirks)
I seem to love everything that can kill me.

                              AARON
That's not funny, Jared.
  What's bothering you?

                              JARED
Nothing, all right?

                              AARON
I thought we were friends.

                              JARED
We are.

AARON

How can we be friends if you won't tell me what's going on?

JARED

Nothing's going on, okay?

AARON

I'm not stupid...Trust me.

(Cyc to Purple)

JARED

Robert!

ROBERT

What?

JARED
(Indicates spot between Jared and Aaron)
Stand there.

ROBERT
(Faces Aaron)
Don't get too close, Aaron. I'm not ready.

AARON

You're putting up walls to stop me? What's bothering you, Jared? Tell me.

JARED

Robin.

(Robin crosses and stands in front of Robert, facing Aaron)

ROBIN
Just stop. I'm not ready to talk.

AARON
I'll break through these walls if you let me.

JARED
Marion.

(Marion crosses and stands in front of Robin, facing Aaron)

MARION
If I wanted you to know what's going on, I'd tell you...

AARON
I'll reach through any obstruction you place between us.

JARED
Helen.

(Helen crosses and stands in front of Marion, facing Aaron)

HELEN
Walls are easy to start, but can never be finished. There cannot be room for a door.

AARON

If only you would open up and talk to me. You have
such strong walls.

JARED

If I let down my walls, I'll be vulnerable.

AARON

We all take that chance, but sometimes it's worth it.

JARED

Will you share my walls?

AARON

Walls are meant to be torn down. Feelings are what
we share.

JARED

I can't handle rejection.

AARON

Let your defenses down...not me.

JARED

I have...

ROBIN

(Faces Jared)

Admit it.

JARED

I have...

ROBERT
(Face Jared)
Tell him.

JARED
I'm sick.

HELEN
(Steps away)
It's a little bit of communication that breaks those
barriers.

JARED
Really sick, and I'm scared.

AARON
I'm here for you.

MARION
(Steps away)
Bonds begin to build.

JARED
I feel so alone.

AARON
I'll never leave.

ROBIN
(Steps away)
A promise made is a breakthrough.

JARED
I have AIDS.

ROBERT
(Steps away)
Trust begins with truth.

AARON
You have what?

(Cyc to white)

JARED
AIDS.

AARON
Why didn't you tell anyone?

JARED
Yeah. Like it's a real ice-breaker. My name is Jared, I like romantic walks on the beach; I'm vegetarian; I have a life-threatening disease, I prefer silk underwear...

AARON
You don't give anyone enough credit.

JARED
I give credit. When you told me about your son...I wanted to bad to tell you that I had AIDS. Me. Your friend...Scared as hell because he has a life-threatening disease that's going to shred him to pieces. I wanted to say, "Aaron...Help me!" But what can you do? What can any of us do? Nothing.

HELEN

We could be here for you.

AARON

Hold you.

JARED

Through latex gloves.

AARON

I'll make sure I never wear gloves when we're together. And, who knows, maybe you'll be the one to beat this, and you'll be the cure.

JARED

Yeah. Right.

ROBIN

I hate those damn latex gloves. It's not like latex can stop AIDS.

ROBERT

Condoms are latex.

ROBIN

But condoms aren't one hundred percent guaranteed.

ROBERT

Some chance of stopping it is better than no chance of stopping it.

JARED

Too late for me.

ROBERT

It's never too late.

JARED

It's already in me. There's no cure.

ROBERT

Maybe they'll start you on AZT or Interferon.

HELEN

Yes. I hear they're making great strides toward a cure.

(Jared picks up empty glass)

JARED

They're going to start me on a strict med regimen, but there's no promises. I'm dying from AIDS. These pills may slow down or stop the virus...

(Jared pours some purple pills (colored candy) into the glass)

ROBIN

(Taking glass from Jared - Pours in Blue Pills)

But you have to take these pills to counteract the bad effects of those pills.

MARION

(Taking glass from Robin - Pours in Green Pills)

And these will help the side-effects of those pills.

ROBERT
(Taking glass from Marion - Pours in Yellow
Pills)
And these which help you sleep.

HELEN
(Taking glass from Robert - Pours in Orange
Pills)
And these which help you stay awake.

AARON
(Taking glass from Helen - Pours in Red
Pills)
And these.

JARED
What are those for?

AARON
Clinical trials.
(Hands FULL glass to Jared)
Cocktail? Now you're living!

(Cyc to white)

JARED
Maybe...just maybe...the drugs will help me beat my
AIDS.

ROBERT
How did you get it?

HELEN
Robert!

ROBERT
Sorry, not to be rude...I was just...

JARED
        (Interrupting)
It's okay...Really.
        (Pause)
My boyfriend died from it.

AARON
What?

ROBIN
You're gay?

AARON
You're my best friend, and you couldn't tell me?

JARED
You hate gays.

AARON
I don't understand them...Oh my God...You've seen
me naked.

HELEN
What?

AARON
In the showers at the gym...What were you
thinking?

JARED

Two six-packs and an ounce and you'd be mine
    (Pause)
What do you mean what did I think? You're my friend and you're straight. I didn't even look...
    (...)
Okay, I looked, but you're off limits...I mean...I didn't even think about it.

MARION

Yeah...sure.

JARED

I didn't.

MARION

Probably lying. That's all men think about. Sex. Sex. Sex.

JARED

The hell with you, Marion. He's my friend. Some of us guys know how to respect friendship.

AARON

Respect it enough to tell your friend the truth?

JARED

I don't want to lose you. You're the only friend I have, anymore. And I'll probably lose you, now. It's just...it's just that...I need a friend.

HELEN

We're all your friends.

JARED
You'll all turn your back on me when...
        (Stops)

ROBERT
When what?

ROBIN
Does this have anything to do with Brent?

AARON
Brent? You're dating Brent?

ROBIN
I asked Brent how he's doing because Jared told us
he has AIDS.

HELEN
Me, too. And Brent was confused.

ROBIN
Brent doesn't have AIDS.

JARED
Okay. Okay. I lied. Brent doesn't have AIDS...
        (Pause)
I wanted to see how you'd all react to someone with
AIDS before I told you about me, and, in a way, you
did.

        (Quick light change to 'inner-thought' mood
        - Quick dialogue)

ROBERT
I didn't really know him... pity.

JARED
Pessimism.

HELEN
Poor boy, he wasn't monogamous.

JARED
Condescending.

ROBIN
I hope he made his peace with God.

JARED
Judgmental.

AARON
A choreographer is a terrible thing to waste.

JARED
Sarcasm.

MARION
Let the faggot die.

JARED
Hatred.
        (Lights back to previous setting)
   I don't want to be alone, and now I'll probably be because none of you know what it's like to know you have this disease, and I pray none of you ever do.

AARON
(Pulls out paper he found on floor earlier)
So...This is yours?

JARED
(Taking paper: reads)
Yes. I'm patient L-0-7-2-6-1-9-8-5.
(soft)
I have AIDS.

(Silence)

HELEN
Is there anything...?

JARED
I just need friends...people to stay by me.

AARON
I'll always be your friend. Always.

(Aaron and Jared hug)

ROBIN
A promise made...

ROBERT
Is a promise until...

HELEN
The end.

                    ROBIN
Where do we go from here?

          (Helen will kneel at casket for a moment. She
          will place two red roses.)

                    HELEN
I wish I knew.

                    JARED
          (Hands Marion the white rose)
A peace offering.

                    MARION
It's yours.

                    JARED
Take it.

          (Marion walks away. Jared sits, holding his
          white rose)

                    ROBERT
          (Approaching Jared)
Jared?

                    JARED
Yeah?

                    ROBERT
I wanted to know...
          (Blurts)
Will you go out with me? On a date? You know:
Dinner, movie, drinks...

JARED

I can't.

ROBERT

Why?

JARED

Robert...I have AIDS.

ROBERT

I know.

JARED

You'll catch it.

ROBERT

From dinner?

JARED

From when we...you know...how do most dates end?

ROBERT

Mine end with a hug, a kiss and a promise to call tomorrow.

JARED

As if. Most end up with someone's legs in the air and a deep pounding...

ROBERT

I'd rather have your hand in mine, and the only pounding be our hearts beating together...

ROBERT

(Continued: Pause - Takes Jared's hand. Jared pulls away. Robert softly grabs his hand)

Look, maybe you've met the wrong guys. Or maybe you just haven't been in the scene that long. I don't know. What I do know is that people who are interested in making a life-long commitment don't think about sex first. They think about the moment they first met...

JARED

(Takes off Robert's black shirt...Robert is wearing a yellow t-shirt)

At auditions for this show...You were wearing that yellow turtleneck. You looked like a penis.

ROBERT

Thank you...

(Removing Jared's black shirt to reveal a purple t-shirt)

And you wore a purple t-shirt...

JARED

You remember? Why?

ROBERT

I think the question would be more, why do *you* remember what I was wearing? You're not like me. I'm out and proud, Jared. I'm gay, and you hide in the closet, but you intrigue me. I do not have AIDS, but I do have a heart.

JARED
And it'll be broken when I die.

ROBERT
Dammit. You can't live waiting to die.

   You being positive for AIDS doesn't make you an outcast. You just have to....well...

   I have a great friend, more like a brother, Vince. He has AIDS. At first, I didn't know what to do, how to handle it, how to be around him...He took the time to teach me the best ways to avoid it. Nothing is one hundred percent guaranteed, but knowing if you have it or not, and educating yourself with current information is the best way to not get it.

JARED
So I'm stupid for catching it?

ROBERT
No. Not at all. No one is stupid for catching this.

   Jared, the one thing you're going to have to learn is that you did not deserve this.

JARED
Yes, I did.

   You know what I did? I went to the bar after my first lover committed suicide and got drunk...The back-bar was closed because someone said you can catch AIDS because of them...That didn't stop me...I dropped my pants, bent over a barstool and let whoever do whatever they wanted.

ROBERT
You were grieving...

JARED

I was guilty. I killed Kevin. He committed suicide because he found out he had AIDS. When I finally...finally went to get tested, you know what the doctor told me? I've had AIDS for seven years. I'm not showing any signs...I'm not losing weight, no splotches on my body...I look clean...God, I hate that term...but me...I killed Kevin and I killed Mark.

ROBERT

You did not kill them...

JARED

I've had AIDS for seven years, Robert. Maybe I'm the carrier. Maybe I'm patient zero.

ROBERT

Maybe you're just one of the lucky ones. AIDS is a death-sentence for many...most people who get it, but not everyone dies in the first year. Some are living long lives naturally.

MARION

Maybe Jared is the one...

ROBERT

Shut up, Marion.

MARION

No...Maybe he is. That's what gays get for what they do. It's what men get for what they do. I mean, how can one man take another man and have sex? It's the most disgusting thing ever.

MARION
(Continued)
That's why I'm a lesbian. Lesbians have always been accepted.

AARON
Not always.

MARION
Oh, please, what straight man out there hasn't fantasized about him and a couple of women playing harem? They think all women want them...But that's men for you, give them an inch and they swear they're hung. Always lying to women, always belittling women...Firing them from jobs if they don't give in.
And then things were made even.
Men get AIDS.
Men are the ones responsible. Not needles. Gay men. They're the cause of all this. If it weren't for men, Nicole wouldn't be sick.

HELEN
Wouldn't be sick? Men don't cause cancer.

MARION
(Stammers)
Men cause all sickness.

(The cast exchanges glances. No one is buying Marion's story anymore.)

ROBERT

It's not just men, Marion. You're always looking for someone to blame. Fine, blame the people out there having unsafe sex...

MARION

Gay men have unsafe sex.

ROBERT

Blame the people using dirty needles.

MARION

Gay men use dirty needles.

ROBERT

What about straight people with dirty needles?

MARION

They're immune.

JARED

What? AIDS doesn't put the brakes on for them.

MARION

Yes, it does. AIDS can distinguish between straight and gay, male or female.

ROBERT

That's a misconception.

MARION

Parents who had gay sons had misconceptions.

HELEN

Hey! Ralph was no misconception. He may not live the life I thought he would...He may never give me a grandchild...but he was never a mistake.

MARION

You're only fooling yourself. Once he comes home with AIDS, you'll wish he was straight.

HELEN

If he comes home and tells me he has AIDS, I'll love him just the same.

ROBERT

Face the truth, Marion, AIDS can hit anyone at any time.

MARION

AIDS is a disease that affects only the people who deserve it, and Nicole didn't deserve it.

HELEN

So she does have AIDS.

MARION

No. She can't. She's a good woman.

JARED

Are you saying I'm a bad man?

MARION

If the shoe fits, homo...

JARED

I'm a bad man because I have AIDS. Aaron's wife was a bad woman because she got AIDS...Aaron's baby is a bad seed because he has AIDS...All those people out there in the world are bad because they caught a disease?

MARION

No, I meant...

JARED

We know what you meant, Marion. Just like all those holier-than-thou's out there, you think you're safe.
    Who you going to turn to if you catch AIDS?

MARION

I was tested...I'm negative. Do you hear me? Negative. I am a woman, and women don't get AIDS.

HELEN

Yes, they do. Marion, I'm going to level with you...woman to woman...Ralph and Gary are buddies to a woman in Whappa, and she has AIDS.

AARON

Buddies?

HELEN

That's what they call them. "Buddies". I guess it makes them feel like friends, without the emotional connection. I don't know. I should join the group.

ROBERT

Yes. Find time to help.

HELEN

Most definitely.

JARED

I talked with Ralph after the show. He told me when he called Gary at intermission; Gary said the woman was feeling really bad tonight...He couldn't go see her because he has the flu, so Ralph was going to be with her.

HELEN

She's been in a lot of pain lately...She has AIDS, Marion...No one is sure how she got it, but she has it. Face it...no one is above this disease, honey...No one.

MARION

But...

HELEN

No one.

MARION

The women who get it were unsafe...They should have made men wear rubbers.

AARON

I didn't give it to my wife...

MARION

Only gay men can give it to a woman.

ROBERT

Sorry, precious, but a gay man wouldn't want a woman.

MARION

Then your wife and that woman must have gotten AIDS from a blood transfusion from a gay man whose blood made it through a window.

(Hands up in triumph)

I found the connection.

(Walks to phone, picks it up, and dials)

ROBIN

Wow. I mean...really...wow.

ROBERT

Some people will never admit the truth. Never. What amazes me is the Lesbian community is the most vocal and extremely active in the fight against AIDS.

ROBIN

Shut up with your lying.

ROBERT

No lie. Lesbians are forming groups to help hold the government accountable, they're telling everyone about safe sex...Lesbians are instrumental in the AIDS struggle...So, to have Marion be so...so...against them and uninformed...Like you said, "wow."

AARON

I told you lesbians were okay in my book.

ROBIN

Don't you even think about starting up, Aaron.

(A group chuckle)

HELEN

We should get back here cleaned up. I hear they're having a party for us...

(Helen motions to Aaron and Robin that Robert and Jared need to talk. As they clean up, Helen, Aaron and Robin will take off their black shirts, revealing that they are wearing t-shirts in their signature color.)

AARON

She's right.

(Everyone except for Robert and Jared will straighten up...unobtrusively so not to distract from Robert and Jared. Marion will hang up phone and go to her seat, taking off her black shirt to show a green t-shirt under.)

ROBERT

Jared? You never answered me.
   Will you go on a date with me?

JARED

No.

ROBERT

Why not?

JARED

I can't stand to think of another person I love going through pain. If you and I end up together, that's all I'll cause you.

ROBERT

Maybe I'll go first, and I'll be the one who is sorry for causing you pain.

JARED

How can you go first? I'm the sick one.

ROBERT

I could walk out of this theatre tonight and get hit by a bus. Tomorrow is not guaranteed for any of us. What is guaranteed is an answer.

You stole my heart the moment we met.

Maybe you and I aren't meant to be together. Maybe we'll never get to that deep-pounding part...but...I mean...what if we are?

What if we're supposed to be together, find a better universe, a better world? Maybe uncover a world where no one knows fear or hatred, find a world where people only know love?

Or maybe all you need is someone who will love you...for you.

All I'm asking for is a chance.

JARED

A chance? That's like finally seeing something you always wanted. Love was all I ever looked for.

When I was a young boy, much younger than you see...I wanted to jump in the ocean; I wanted to swim in the sea. But those waters are for big boys, and I wasn't one to know, but in the future days of life; sailing those seas, I would go. I'm older now and dying. I wallowed those waters along the way. My illusions are now dead within them; our destiny join together on a not too distant day.

(Hands Robert the white rose)
What if I give you AIDS?

ROBERT

(Hands rose back)
What if you don't?

(Slowly moves in to kiss Jared. Jared pulls back. Robert relents)
Maybe, just maybe, you'll give me a new life. My chance to swim in the ocean.

And, baby, you're not dead yet. That ocean may be calling you to take another swim.

You've seen your ocean...You've had a chance to feel its waters embrace you. Me? I've never known real love. I've never had that one person in my life. I've had a lot of people in my life...Few had names, hell, some didn't even have faces...Does that mean I don't deserve happiness somewhere in the game?

JARED

You love me?

ROBERT

Hell if I know, Jared. But before we start picking out wedding chapels...why don't we explore being friends?

JARED

What if we fall in love?

ROBERT

Then we'll fall in love.

JARED

I'm scared.

ROBERT

Would you rather be scared alone, or in the arms of someone?

JARED

I do like you.

ROBERT

Then we're halfway there.

JARED

(Pause)
Yes, Robert...I'll go on a date with you.

(SOUND: Phone Ring)

AARON

Probably the stage manager telling us to hurry up. They love to leave as soon as everything is set for the next performance.

(Robin races Marion to phone, wins, and answers)

ROBIN

Helen? It's your son.

HELEN
(Grabs phone)
Ralph?...Is Gary alright?
(Everyone stops and looks at Helen)
...Are you sure?...Wait...Who?...You're certain?...
Okay, honey....I'll...I'll talk to you soon.
(Hangs up phone)

ROBERT

Is everything okay?

HELEN

Marion? Honey? Marion?

MARION

Yeah?

HELEN
(Crosses to Marion)
Your friend, Nicole, just passed away.

MARION

What?

HELEN

Nicole died, honey. About five minutes ago. Ralph was at her side, and she told him...

MARION
(Slaps Helen - or Aaron - depending on Helen's physical make up)
Shut up. Just shut up.

HELEN
She said she loves you and she's sorry that her AIDS was stronger than both of you.

(Cyc to Green)

MARION
She didn't have AIDS. Women don't get AIDS.

ROBIN
What is it going to take to get through to you, Marion? Women can get it.

AARON
Straights can get it.

ROBERT
Gays can get it.

JARED
I can get it.

MARION
Nicole was never one to stop fighting. I was. Look what she did to me.
I'm alone, dammit, alone! And it's all her fault. She can't be dead. She can't.

MARION
(Continued)
Your son was wrong. It wasn't Nicole. Cancer.
That's all she had. Don't let my emotions fool you.
Cancer. Nicole died from cancer.
How would he even know to call here?

JARED
I told him at intermission. I said I think the woman
they're with is Nicole. He was going to check her
wristband

MARION
Why? I told you she only has cancer.
When she went into the hospital, I knew she was
in the wrong area. They did a total hysterectomy.
They got it all. I promised God I'd be good if He took
it all away. And He did. I was good. Why did He
break His promise?

HELEN
She didn't die from cancer. No promise was broken.

MARION
(Crying as Helen comforts her...This is not an
angry moment)
Yes, she did.

HELEN
Nicole had AIDS, sweetie. AIDS.

MARION
No. Why my Nicole?

ROBIN

There's no "why"...She didn't do anything wrong, baby. None of these people who have AIDS did anything wrong.

MARION

Oh my God...My heart is gone.

HELEN

(Cradling Marion)
Hush, sweetie...
(Comforting)
Don't throw away the beautiful memories you and Nicole shared by disrespecting her death. If you do that, Nicole becomes another nameless statistic. Proudly declare that she was a warrior in the fight against AIDS, and AIDS may have defeated her battle, but it has not defeated us all.

MARION

But what am I going to do? What can any of us do? We're helpless against a virus. I wanted to believe that it couldn't get to all of us...but it can. It's the end of the world.

HELEN

Not all of us will get it.

MARION

But why did I believe women can't get it?

HELEN

Because you needed to believe it, but your truths...your truth.

ROBIN

The mirror got twisted. Marion. My brother, straight as an arrow and clean as a whistle, got AIDS. Not saying people with AIDS is dirty, but, everyone can get it. He got it. Aaron's little one got it, and didn't do nothing wrong. Aaron's wife died from it, and she was a woman. What more do you need to understand that AIDS affects everyone?

MARION

I don't want to believe it. I can't. If I believe that, then it makes AIDS real.

ROBERT

AIDS is real.

JARED

You can't wish it away.

MARION

I don't want it here. I want it to go away. I don't want anyone else to die.

AARON

No one else should have to die.

MARION

That's what the sisterhood preached.

ROBIN

The sisterhood?

MARION

A lesbian group...That's where I met Nicole. On one
of their bike rallies.

ROBERT

I like bicycles.

MARION

Harleys, Ducatis, Kawasakis, gay boy.

ROBERT

Ah...Lesbian vibrators.

MARION

Real women respect the road.
   I saw her sitting on a rice-burner, and had to save
her, and she ended up saving me. We travelled this
country together on those bike rides. Act up: Stop
AIDS. Bring awareness and attention...Do whatever
we could to stop this AIDS thing. Silence equals
death.
   Then she met my boss. Nicole liked men, too, and
she really liked James. Here we are dating, and she's
screwing my boss. Thing was, he was a druggie...

AARON

Sorry.

MARION

She never stuck a needle in her arm...but...well...One

MARION
(Continued)

night, my boss was really high, and he and Nicole were doing it right there on our bed. My bed...and then I walk in and he wants me to join. To hell with that. He fired me the next day. Died six months later.

ROBERT

That was awful quick. Didn't he show any signs?

MARION

He didn't know he was infected until after he was with Nicole. That's what's scary about AIDS. Sometimes it never shows up.

When Nicole tested positive, she told him. He tests, finds out he has it. Kills himself when people started telling him they didn't know he was gay. Even I starting thinking he was gay.

Only gay men get the disease.

We did bike rides and they called us Dykes on Bikes. Different groups, but nationally, one club. We stopped in gay bars. We went to gay community centers. There's even a gay church now, and they have AIDS outreach. Everywhere we rallied, it was a gay group. All the signs point to AIDS being a gay disease.

ROBERT

The gay community embraced the cause. Sure, straight people are getting it, but AIDS is predominant in our life. Everyone else had the chance to say, "Whew! It's not us!", but the gay community never got that break. The finger pointed straight at us.

ROBERT

(Continued)

We started fighting the disease from day one.

MARION

God, how could I be so stupid? Fighting a disease I don't really know anything about.

ROBERT

What do you know about it?

MARION

Not much. It kills. It hurts. It breaks hearts.

ROBERT

And?

MARION

People dying from AIDS need understanding, compassion and love.

ROBIN

Then learn to understand.

MARION

I will.

AARON

Learn to care.

MARION

I will.

JARED

And, above it all...Never stop the love.

MARION

Never.
        (Pause)
I don't know what I'm going to do.

JARED

You're going to be strong. You're going to face the truth, and you're going to continue living.

MARION

I can't even afford her funeral. We wasted so much money on tests and treatment. Insurance doesn't cover...

JARED

        (Interrupting)
I have some money saved up. I'll help you with the expenses.

MARION

You're going to need that money for you.

JARED

I'll be fine.

MARION

I said some nasty shit to you.

JARED

It's in the past. You need help...I'm here for you.

MARION

I'm so sorry I said...

JARED

Don't...

MARION
(Breaks down crying - releases hold on rose)
Oh, my God...Nicole is dead.

JARED

I know...I'm sorry.

MARION

She died...

JARED

Yes.

MARION

She wasn't lying to me.

JARED

No.

MARION
(Holds rose with Jared again)
As God as my witness, and in front of everyone, I vow to do everything in my power to kill the disease that's killed Nicole...that's killed so many.

   Nicole died today...She was a woman, a lesbian, my lover and...She...She had AIDS.

(AFTER Marion's line, Jared and Marion place the white rose on the casket and step away.)

(Cyc to white)

(Marion steps forward, directly to audience)

MARION

But, even after all that, will anyone listen? We can learn and care and love...but where do we go from here?
(Pause)
Seriously? Where do we go from here? There's no roadmap. There's no end in sight. We just kick the starter and point the pig at the horizon? I rode in defiance, in hope, in love...and our destination was...nowhere? How many more people have to die? Where do we go from here?

HELEN

Where do we go from here? I wish I knew. I do know that I'm scared, but I have to trust that people are safe. I have to hope that they remain safe, but I know I will love them until the day I...well...the day after forever ends. I think that's the answer, but I'm not sure. I mean...Where do we go from here?

AARON

Where do we go from here? I asked that so many times. My son will leave me, and my wife is already gone. She's up there, protecting us...I hope you know that...She's one of the angels now...Maybe

MARION

(Continued)

that's where we go...Maybe it isn't...I don't know. Where do we go from here?

ROBERT

Where do we go from here? What a laugh. I sit and think about me and Vince sometimes, and I try to make sense of it all. We were both, well, not the safest people out there. If I get AIDS, I want someone there to hold my hand. Maybe that's the answer, being there for someone, or someone being there for you. I hope it is, if it's not...then where do we go from here?

ROBIN

Where do we go from here? When I found out Brian had AIDS, you know what I did? I thanked God it wasn't me. Now I pray to God that Brian would get well and I could get sick instead. I think everyone who knows someone with AIDS blames themselves, and that needs to stop. Maybe forgiveness is the reason...I forgive you, Brian, for taking away my sins...I will live for you, and because of you, but where do we go from here?

JARED

Where do we go from here? I have this damn disease, it's killing me, and there's nothing I can do to stop it. I won't give up...I will hold onto that small part of me that hopes an answer is out there. Sometimes a fantasy comes true. Maybe that's where we go...Maybe we find the dream. Maybe we

JARED
(Continued)
hold the fantasy. Maybe we've had the answer all
along, and just haven't noticed it.
(Softly, pointing out over audience)
Look, a unicorn.

(The cast back into character - fourth wall
back up. Stage Manager enters)

STAGE MANAGER
Stage is set. Time to call it a night.

HELEN
Marion's partner passed away.

STAGE MANAGER
I'm sorry.

JARED
Too many people dying. Too many people suffering.

ROBIN
Looks like we're all angels that didn't protect those
they love. We are the fallen guardian angels we
feared would appear tonight.

MARION
Fuck a monkey! I am not fallen! We are not fallen,
Robin, none of us. As Nicole has often said, as my
sisters on the road have often said: We are warriors
in this fight, too!

ROBIN
Then who are the fallen?

ROBERT
Not us.
(To Stage Manager)
Right? Or are we the fallen?

(Cyc out. Marion grabs a flameless candle.
She turns on the light, and places it at one
end of the casket. For simplicity, when the
action simply states "Character: Light" - the
named character will also light a similar
flameless candle and place it in front of the
casket..)

STAGE MANAGER
We cannot be the fallen
(Marion: Light)
when we walk this earth looking for the lost and
orphaned to bring them back home with soft
heartfelt words.
We cannot be fallen
(Jared: Light)
searching all others to discover their hidden pain,
and ease it away with a loving hold.
We are not fallen
(Robert: Light)
when fighting for respect for those unable to fight
for themselves in an ugly world.
Are we considered fallen
(Aaron: Light)
for casting barriers aside from holding love in
tarnished cages away from others?

STAGE MANAGER

(Continued)

Why call us fallen

(Helen: Light)

when we accept the truth while breaking evil lies of
hate and relinquishing their grip over us as we deny
what they believe so dear?

We are not fallen

(Robin: Light)

wanting true justice for those cast aside by a vile
hatred branded on them for doing nothing wrong.

(Cyc soft white)

We are not fallen...We are not to blame.

JARED

But what do we do?

HELEN

Is there anything we can do?

STAGE MANAGER

We do what has to be done. It's the responsible thing
to do.

ROBIN

But all we ever hear is people saying the ball's not in
their park.

AARON

I don't think the ball is in one person's park.

HELEN

It's everywhere.

ROBERT
And it's not going to go away without a fight.

MARION
It's time we unite.

AARON
One solid force.

JARED
And conquer this damn thing...together.

ALL
(To audience)
Where do we go from here?

(Robin, determined, takes center stage after a
pause.)

ROBIN
We find hope, and we move onward.

AARON
We find a voice, and move onward!

HELEN
We find love, and move onward!

ROBERT
We find heart, and move onward!

JARED
We find forgiveness, and move onward!

MARION

We find truth, and move onward!

STAGE MANAGER

The door is open. Welcome back to today. To what we discovered over the years. How HIV spreads, how to control the disease, how it inhabits the blood, and not kill it, and how to protect ourselves. We now know it's not just a gay disease. We're back, and once we step through that door; we leave our illusions behind, reality rears its ugly head, and complacency takes hold if we do nothing.

Do what you can. Speak up. Act out. Silence will ultimately lead to death.

Be strong. Be proud. Be compassion.

And be love.

So I ask you...

Where do we go from here?

> (As they say their next line, each cast member will step to the front of the stage, their colors in order - Red to purple - and hold their fist up in defiance)

AARON

We go forward and
           (Raises fist now)
onward!

HELEN

Onward!

ROBERT

Onward!

MARION

Onward!

ROBIN

Onward!

JARED

Onward!

ALL

Until *we* find the answer.

> (The lights fade. Suggestion: At some point
> during act two after the "costume change",
> Aaron had tossed his red tie on top of the
> casket. At one point while the Stage Manager
> spoke of the open doors, Aaron discreetly
> fashions the tie to look like an HIV/AIDS
> awareness ribbon and not fully exposed until
> after curtain calls. Although the Red Ribbon
> campaign did not begin until 1991, the Stage
> Manager has brought us back to the present,
> so it would not be an anachronism)

END ACT TWO

END OF PLAY

Fallen Guardian Angels